ECAT Assay Procedures

A Manual of Laboratory Techniques

ECAT Assay Procedures
A Manual of Laboratory Techniques

European Concerted Action on Thrombosis and Disabilities of the Commission of the European Communities

Edited by
J. Jespersen
Department of Clinical Chemistry
Ribe County Hospital in Esbjerg
Esbjerg, Denmark

R. M. Bertina
Haemostasis and Thrombosis Research Unit
University Hospital, Leiden
Leiden, The Netherlands

F. Haverkate
IVVO-TNO
Gaubius Laboratory
Leiden, The Netherlands

 SPRINGER SCIENCE+BUSINESS MEDIA, B.V.

British Library Cataloguing in Publication Data

ECAT assay procedures : a manual of laboratory techniques
I. Jespersen, J. II. Bertina, R. M. (Rogier M)
III. Haverkate, F.
616.135

ISBN 978-94-010-5330-3

Library of Congress Cataloging in Publication Data

ECAT assay procedures: a manual of laboratory techniques/European Concerted Action on
   Thrombosis and Disabilities of the Commission of the European Communities; edited by
   J. Jespersen, R. M. Bertina, F. Haverkate.
       p. cm.
   Includes bibliographical references and index.
   ISBN 978-94-010-5330-3   ISBN 978-94-011-2992-3 (eBook)
   DOI 10.1007/978-94-011-2992-3
   1. Blood coagulation tests. 2. Thrombosis—Risk factors. 3. Thrombosis—Diagnosis.
I. Jespersen, Jørgen. II. Bertina, Rogier M. III. Haverkate, F. (Frits), 1931– . IV. European
Concerted Action on Thrombosis and Disabilities (Committee). V. Commission of the
European Communities.
       [DNLM: 1. Diagnosis, Laboratory—methods. 2. Hemostatics—analysis—laboratory manuals.
   3. Thrombosis—blood—laboratory manuals. QY 25 E17]
   RB45.3.E23   1992
   616.07'561—dc20
   DNLM/DLC
   for Library of Congress   91-46718
                                                                                  CIP

Typeset by Technical Keying Services, Manchester.

Contents

Preface

This book offers a description of current and recently developed laboratory assays in the field of haemostasis and thrombosis. It is the result of a unique cooperation between experts from more than 60 institutes in 12 European countries, brought together by the ECAT (European Concerted Action on Thrombosis and Disabilities) under the auspices of the Commission of the European Communities in Brussels, Belgium.

The ECAT, which was initiated in 1981, designed and performed three prospective clinical studies to establish haemostatic factors as risk indicators of thrombosis. Included were patients with angina pectoris at risk from myocardial infarction, patients undergoing angioplasty at risk from re-stenosis, and patients receiving hip replacement at risk from deep venous thrombosis. Assay procedures were chosen, training courses for technicians held, and essential reagents were supplied from a central source. A quality control assessment scheme served to compare assay results both within and between laboratories. In the angina pectoris study, centres determined most of the assays locally; in the other two studies assays were performed centrally. The need for further quality assessment in Europe led to a separate activity coordinated by Dr J. F. Davidson in Glasgow, including coagulation inhibitors and plasminogen as risk factors for familial venous thrombosis. The Editors hope the *ECAT Assay Procedures* book will contribute to further harmonization of haemostasis assays, and ultimately to their standardization. The need for this is evident from the failure of the ECAT quality controls to demonstrate an obvious improvement in the agreement in haemostasis assay results between laboratories.

This book has been preceded by two editions produced for internal use only. Each assay was assessed by an expert who functioned in the ECAT as representative of a reference laboratory. An assay committee coordinated the activities. Each chapter in this book is written by the assay expert. Most of the chapters give a detailed description of the assay recommended for use in ECAT and briefly mention alternatives. For this reason we have included a list of firms marketing kits and reagents at the back of the book. The Editors will be happy to receive critical comments, as well as suggestions for reagents and assays. They can be included in the next updated version which will be prepared as soon as the need arises.

The Editors are indebted to the Commission of the European Communities, to all ECAT participants who directly or indirectly were of great value, and in particular to Professor F. Duckert, Basel, who did most of the pioneering work.

Esbjerg, Leiden, 1991   **Jørgen Jespersen**
                                                        Rogier Bertina
                                                        Frits Haverkate

List of Contributors

M. C. ALESSI MD PhD
Laboratoire Hématologie
University Hospital, La Timone
Marseilles
France

ROGIER M. BERTINA PhD
Haemostasis and Thrombosis Research
Unit
University Hospital Leiden
Leiden
The Netherlands

A. BINDER PhD
Technoclone Ltd.
Vienna
Austria

BERND R. BINDER MD
Laboratory for Clinical Experimental
Physiology
University of Vienna
Austria

JACQUELINE CONARD PhD
Laboratoire Central d'Hématologie
Hotel-Dieu
Paris
France

PETER C. COOPER
Department of Haematology
Royal Hallamshire Hospital
Sheffield
UK

R. COPPOLA PhD
A. Bianchi Bonomi Hemophilia and
Thrombosis Center and Institute of Internal
Medicine
University of Milano
Milano
Italy

FRANÇOIS DUCKERT Dr ès Sc Dr med h c
Coagulation Laboratory
Kontonsspital Basel
Basel
Switzerland

PATRICK J. GAFFNEY PhD DSc
National Institute for Biological Standards
and Control
Potters Bar
London
UK

JØRGEN GRAM MD DSc
Department of Clinical Chemistry
Ribe County Hospital in Esbjerg
Esbjerg
Denmark

ANDRÉ HAEBERLI PhD
Department of Medicine
University of Bern
Inselspital
Bern
Switzerland

JOB HARENBERG MD PhD
1st Department of Medicine
Faculty of Clinical Medicine Mannheim
University of Heidelberg
Klinikum Mannheim
Mannheim
Germany

E. HATTEY BScI
Laboratory for Clinical Experimental
Physiology
University of Vienna
Austria

M. HAUMER
Laboratory for Clinical Experimental
Physiology
University of Vienna
Austria

F. HAVERKATE MD
IVVO-TNO
Gaubius Laboratory
Leiden
The Netherlands

JØRGEN JESPERSEN MD DSc
Department of Clinical Chemistry
Ribe County Hospital in Esbjerg
Esbjerg
Denmark

IRENE JUHAN-VAGUE MD PhD
Laboratoire Hématologie
University Hospital, La Timone
Marseilles
France

CORNELIS KLUFT PhD
IVVO TNO
Gaubius Laboratory
Leiden
The Netherlands

EGBERT K. O. KRUITHOF PhD
Hematology Laboratory
Department of Medicine
University Hospital
Lausanne
Switzerland

PIER M. MANNUCCI MD PhD
A. Bianchi Bonomi Hemophilia and
Thrombosis Center and Institute of Internal
Medicine
University of Milano
Milano
Italy

GERMAN A. MARBET MD
Coagulation Laboratory
Kantonsspital Basel
Basel
Switzerland

WILLEM NIEUWENHUIZEN PhD
IVVO TNO
Gaubius Laboratory
Leiden
The Netherlands

DUNCAN S. PEPPER PhD
Scottish National Blood Transfusion
Service
Headquarters Laboratory
Edinburgh
UK

LEON POLLER MD DSc
UK Reference Laboratory for Anticoagulant
Reagents and Control
Withington Hospital
Manchester
UK

F. ERIC PRESTON MD
Department of Haematology
Royal Hallamshire Hospital
Sheffield
UK

CHRISTOPHER V. PROWSE PhD
Scottish National Blood Transfusion
Service
National Science Laboratory
Edinburgh
UK

SIMON G. THOMPSON MA
Medical Statistics Unit
London School of Hygiene and Tropical
Medicine
London
UK

JEAN M. THOMSON PhD
UK Reference Laboratory for Anticoagulant
Reagents and Control
Withington Hospital
Manchester
UK

A. TRIPODI PhD
A. Bianchi Bonomi Hemophilia and
Thrombosis Center and Institute of Internal
Medicine
University of Milano
Milano
Italy

JAN H. VERHEIJEN PhD
IVVO TNO
Gaubius Laboratory
Leiden
The Netherlands

1
Quality assessment of haemostatic assays

S. G. THOMPSON and J. M. THOMSON

INTRODUCTION

In order to obtain reproducible results, haemostatic factor assays need to be performed with considerable care. Internal quality control procedures are therefore particularly important in this area of laboratory work. Furthermore, when a group of laboratories are collaborating together in one study, the agreement on results between laboratories also needs to be assessed by an appropriate external quality assessment (QA) scheme. Such was the situation in the ECAT prospective studies, in which different European laboratories performed a range of haemostatic factor assays on patients recruited in their own centres. In the ECAT Deep Vein Thrombosis Study and the ECAT Angioplasty Study most of the assays were performed centrally, but in the ECAT Angina Pectoris Study the majority of assays were performed locally. This chapter therefore, as an example, describes the organization and results of the more extensive QA exercises carried out during the ECAT Angina Pectoris Study[1,2].

The principle of external QA schemes is that identical samples are distributed to all participating laboratories; the results from each laboratory are then compared. Sometimes target values can be defined for QA samples; for example international standards for some of the ECAT assays are available. However, as in the present case, assessment often relies on 'consensus comparison', that is comparison of the results of each laboratory with the average achieved by all. The detailed arrangements for an external QA scheme of course depends on its specific purpose; in the present case this was to establish and maintain quality of performance for the multicentre ECAT Angina Pectoris Study. The aim was to ensure that plasma samples were analysed in a way that was acceptable for a multicentre study, while remaining feasible in each laboratory. The purpose was therefore not to impose fully standardized procedures in each laboratory, but to assess

1

realistically the quality of routine performance and achieve better harmonization of the assay results.

DESIGN OF THE QA EXERCISES

The QA exercises were designed to assess reproducibility of results in three ways, that is between duplicates, between days and between laboratories. The first two of these represent aspects of laboratory performance which can be tested internally by each laboratory. However, an external QA scheme obviously provides additional stimulus to improve performance. Moreover, if one laboratory has poor agreement with others on their assay results, the availability of information on between-duplicate and between-day reproducibility may help in identifying and rectifying problems speedily. In order to establish good performance of the assays as quickly as possible for the ECAT Angina Pectoris Study, these aspects of reproducibility were therefore assessed in the QA exercises.

Five QA exercises were carried out at 6–9 month intervals, over a period of $2\frac{1}{2}$ years. Up to 16 laboratories participated in each one. In each exercise, vials of lyophilized plasmas, numbered 0–9, were prepared from five test plasma pools at the UK Reference Laboratory in Manchester and dispatched by post to each participating laboratory. The samples numbered 5–9 were identical to those numbered 0–4, but the correspondence between the sets varied between exercises and was not revealed to the participating laboratories. Assays were performed in duplicate on each numbered sample. For each assay, samples 0–4 were assayed on one day while samples 5–9 were assayed on a different day.

LABORATORY ARRANGEMENTS

Ten assays were included in each of the five QA exercises. Three of these were based on a clotting procedure (factor VIII:C, fibrinogen [Clauss technique] and activated partial thromboplastin time [APTT]), four on determination of antigen by Laurell rocket immunoelectrophoresis (von Willebrand factor-related antigen [vWF R:Ag], antithrombin III [AT III:Ag], protein C and histidine-rich glycoprotein [HRG]) and three on determination of activity using synthetic chromogenic substrates (antithrombin III [AT III:C], plasminogen and α_2-antiplasmin).

At least one technician from each participating laboratory attended 1-week ECAT training courses, including one on coagulation and one on fibrinolysis assays. The aim of these courses was to establish uniformity in blood collection and laboratory methodology, to extend and consolidate the technicians' existing knowledge, and to make them aware of potential sources of error.

All participating laboratories were circulated with recommended assay procedures, of which this present book is an extended and updated version. Also, certain reagents and kits were distributed centrally: APTT reagent (together with a recommended technique) was supplied by L. Poller, antisera against vWF and AT III by F. Duckert, against protein C by R. M. Bertina, and against HRG by Behringwerke. KabiVitrum provided S-2251 and Kabikinase for the plasminogen assay, and kits for the α_2-antiplasmin and AT III:C assays. It was compulsory to use a one-stage assay for VIII:C and heparin activation for AT III:C. However, the participating laboratories were allowed to use equipment and minor assay modifications of their choice. The establishing of reference curves and the dilution of samples were performed as in routine work in each laboratory, to remain as close as possible to local practice.

Plasmas for external QA must fulfil certain criteria in order to satisfy requirements for their suitability. These include checks on inter-vial variation and long-term stability which were carried out at the production centre following lyophilization, prior to dispatch. When the plasmas were received by the laboratories, they were stored at $-20\,°C$ or lower until required. Each single vial was reconstituted with 1.0 ml of sterile distilled water, then gently mixed, and left at room temperature for 3–5 min to ensure complete reconstitution. Apart from the separate batching of the samples numbered 0–4 and those numbered 5–9, no special instructions were given to laboratories about the assaying of QA samples, for example whether they were to be undertaken by one or several technicians, or whether alone or together with other samples.

Fibrinogen results were expressed in grams per litre and APTT in seconds. Except for these, results were expressed as a percentage of that of a local standard made in each laboratory. The local standard was prepared as a plasma pool from at least 20 normal healthy people, divided into small aliquots in polypropylene tubes for daily use, snap-frozen at less than $-50\,°C$ and subsequently stored at less than $-40\,°C$. Sufficient local standard was made in each laboratory to last the duration of the ECAT Angina Pectoris Study. Since there could be differences in the potencies of the local standards, the *absolute* values obtained by different laboratories could not be directly compared. However, using the *ratios* of duplicate values, or of values obtained on different days, provides a measure of reproducibility which is not affected by the absolute level of results. Similarly, agreement between laboratories could be judged by the *relative* values obtained on the five different plasmas.

PRESENTATION OF RESULTS

It was necessary to provide a synopsis of the results to each laboratory in a form which (1) was easily understood, (2) enabled comparison of their results to those of other laboratories, and (3) maintained confidentiality. The following graphical presentation was the principal method adopted.

The ratios of duplicate values obtained for each of 10 QA samples (numbered 0–9) were calculated for each assay and each laboratory. These ratios were displayed as in Figure 1.1, which shows results for AT III:C, above a different position on the horizontal axis for each laboratory. In such figures a letter code was used to identify laboratories, each laboratory only being told its own code. Ratios close to 1.0 reflect close duplicate results and

3

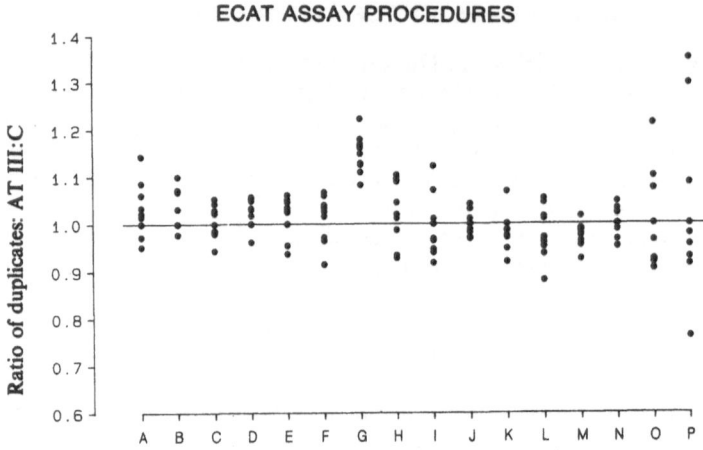

Figure 1.1 Ratios of 10 duplicate pairs of antithrombin III:C values for 16 laboratories in the first QA exercise. (Some points are superimposed)

good performance, while ratios far from 1.0 indicate large differences between duplicates and poor performance. In Figure 1.1, for example, laboratory P showed the poorest results for AT III:C while laboratory J showed good between-duplicate variability.

In order to assess between-day variability, similar graphs were constructed for the ratios of the results on each sample numbered 0–4 to the corresponding sample out of those numbered 5–9. (The result on each sample was taken as the geometric mean of the duplicate determinations.) For AT III:C for example (Figure 1.2), poor between-day reproducibility was evident for laboratories L, M and P.

The first stage in assessing agreement between laboratories was to obtain a measure of the potency of each local standard. For each assay separately,

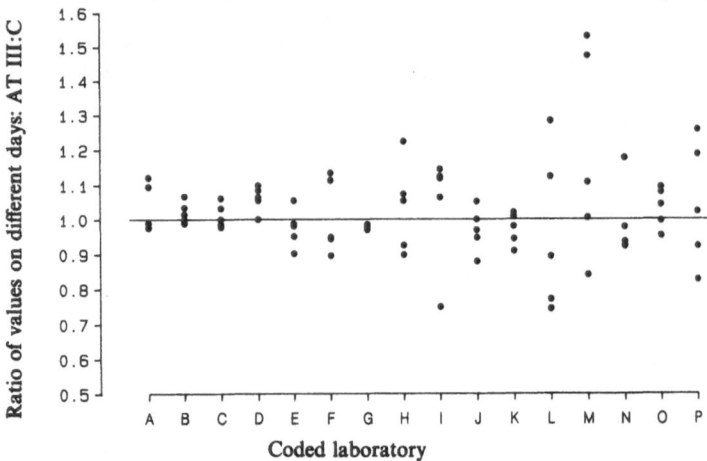

Figure 1.2 Ratios of five antithrombin III:C values in the first QA exercise obtained on different days for 16 laboratories in the first QA exercise. (Some points are superimposed)

therefore, the geometric mean of all the results on all the QA samples was calculated for each laboratory. This overall mean would be high if the local standard had low potency, and vice-versa. For each of the five QA plasmas, each laboratory obtained four results (duplicate determinations on each of two days), and the ratio of the geometric mean of these four results to the overall mean obtained by the laboratory was calculated. These ratios were displayed as in Figure 1.3, with points corresponding to each of the five plasmas joined. Ideally, such a graph should reveal five horizontal straight lines. For AT III:C (Figure 1.3), there is fair separation between the samples' relative values and substantial (though not perfect) agreement between laboratories.

Each laboratory received, in addition to copies of such graphs and a commentary on their interpretation, a confidential synopsis of the possible problems revealed in their own laboratory.

SOME STATISTICAL ISSUES

For the ratios in Figure 1.1, for example, a ratio of 0.8 could be obtained if the first duplicate value was 80% and the second 100%. If the duplicate values were simply reversed, the ratio would be 1.25. Thus a ratio of 0.8 is as 'bad' as a ratio of $1/0.80 = 1.25$, rather than one of 1.2. Similarly a ratio of 0.5 is as bad as a ratio of 2.0, not of 1.5. Hence the most appropriate vertical scale in Figure 1.1 would be a proportionate (i.e. logarithmic) scale, rather than the absolute scale shown. Although for simplicity a log scale was not adopted in practice, this explains why geometric means, rather than the more usual arithmetic means, were used in the calculations.

It is useful to be able to summarize the results, such as those presented in Figure 1.1–1.3, more concisely. Three coefficients of variation (CVs) can in

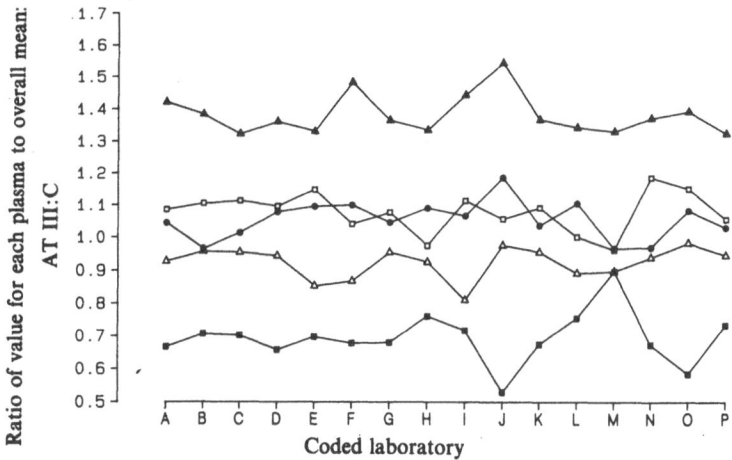

Figure 1.3 Mean antithrombin III:C values for each of five plasmas, expressed relative to their overall geometric mean within each of 16 laboratories in the first QA exercise. Lines join points corresponding to the same plasma

5

fact be calculated for each laboratory, as described in the Appendix, giving measures of between-duplicate, between-day and between-laboratory variability. In line with the preceding comments, these CVs are based on the logarithms of the ratios. If a laboratory shows poor between-duplicate variability it will also tend to show poor between-day variability by virtue of this alone. This is because each sample's result on a particular day is the mean of duplicate determinations. In a statistical sense the between-duplicate and between-day CVs calculated are therefore not independent of each other. Similarly the between-laboratory CV includes components associated with the between-day and between-duplicate variabilities. In Figure 1.3 the geometric mean of the five ratios for each laboratory is unity. So there are only four, not five, independent ratios on which a CV can be based; this is reflected in the formula for the between-laboratory CV (see Appendix).

In general terms, high CVs represent poor performance and low CVs good performance. However, single extreme results can have a dramatic effect on a calculated CV. Thus a CV should not be calculated without inspection of the individual ratios on which it is based. Also, since each CV is based on only five or 10 ratios, they cannot be sensibly interpreted individually. Their use is more to describe the performance of an assay (averaged over laboratories), or of a laboratory (averaged over assays). An assay with high laboratory CVs may be disadvantaged in clinical or epidemiological studies, but should not necessarily be abandoned: the measurement may represent some underlying characteristic which has great enough prognostic importance still to be useful. However, any laboratory with high CVs relative to other laboratories is necessarily hindering a successful outcome to the study; its quality of assay performance is demonstrably poor and should be improved.

RESULTS AND THEIR INTERPRETATION

The calculated CVs for each laboratory for the first QA exercise, averaged over the 10 assays, are shown in Table 1.1 together with their corresponding ranking. Some laboratories showed particular problems in the between-day variability, with high CVs. It is also clear that laboratories which performed poorly according to one measure of variability also tended to perform poorly according to others. Thus the total rank, summed across the three measures of variability, provides a useful summary of the relative performance of each laboratory. There is clearly no sensible way of defining an absolute level of performance to be deemed 'acceptable'. However, those laboratories with the poorest performance (a total rank of greater than 30 in Table 1.1) were not allowed to start analysing patient samples in the ECAT Angina Pectoris Study, until the laboratory problems had been resolved and their results in a future QA exercise had proved more satisfactory. The simple comparison with other laboratories' results was alone a strong stimulus for improvement. These laboratories were also offered discussion with experts, site visits and repeat QA material.

The sequence of five QA exercises provided an insight into the assays for which improvements in performance could be made. The between-duplicate

6

Table 1.1 Mean coefficients of variation (CVs) in the first QA exercise for 16 different laboratories, averaged over 10 assays, with the ranking of CVs and total rank

Coded laboratory	Between-duplicate CV (%)	Rank	Between-day CV (%)	Rank	Between-laboratory CV (%)	Rank	Total rank
A	5.5	13	7.9	10	4.9	3	26
B	4.4	8	5.6	4	5.6	5	17
C	2.7	2	7.2	7	4.2	2	11
D	3.1	4	3.3	1	4.2	1	6
E	3.0	3	4.2	3	6.4	8	14
F	4.8	10	5.7	5	6.0	6	21
G	8.0	16	9.7	11	7.8	12	39
H	4.2	7	7.5	9	7.6	11	27
I	1.8	1	7.1	6	5.1	4	11
J	4.5	9	7.3	8	6.8	9	26
K	3.8	6	3.6	2	6.1	7	15
L	5.8	14	13.9	14	12.6	16	44
M	5.2	11	12.7	12	9.9	14	37
N	3.2	5	17.3	16	7.0	10	31
O	5.3	12	13.0	13	7.9	13	38
P	7.2	15	16.0	15	12.0	15	45

CV for the 10 assays (averaged across the 15 laboratories with continued participation in the QA exercises) is shown in Figure 1.4. The overall average CV decreased consistently from 4.4% in the first QA exercise to 3.2% in the fifth, the trend of improvement being fairly consistent among the 10 assays. APTT in particular, and fibrinogen and plasminogen assays also, showed consistently lower between-duplicate CVs than the other assays.

A similar pattern of improvement was evident overall for the between-day CV (Figure 1.5). Again the APTT assay had the lowest CV in all the exercises, but the extreme differences between the assays for the first two exercises became smaller later on. The initial differences were caused in particular by poor between-day reproducibility for the VIII assays (vWF R:Ag and VIII:C) and AT III:Ag. That improvements were evident in both the between-duplicate and the between-day CVs of course indicates that the QA scheme had, at least to an extent, achieved its purpose.

However, the between-laboratory CV showed no consistent improvement over the five QA exercises (Figure 1.6). Some assays retained low between-laboratory CVs (e.g. APTT) and some high (e.g. α_2-antiplasmin); some showed a reduction in CV (e.g. vWF R:Ag) over the five exercises, but others an increase (e.g. HRG). So while the trends of the CVs differed between the assays, the net effect of these changes was small. The fact that the between-laboratory CV did not improve, despite improvements in the between-duplicate and between-day CVs, is somewhat surprising. It must be due to greater sources of technical variability being incorporated into the comparison between laboratories, for example due to the use of different equipment and minor assay modifications in different laboratories. It is notable that the APTT assay, the only test to be performed with a common reagent and standardized technique, had the lowest between-laboratory CV. The failure to demonstrate an improvement in the agreement between

7

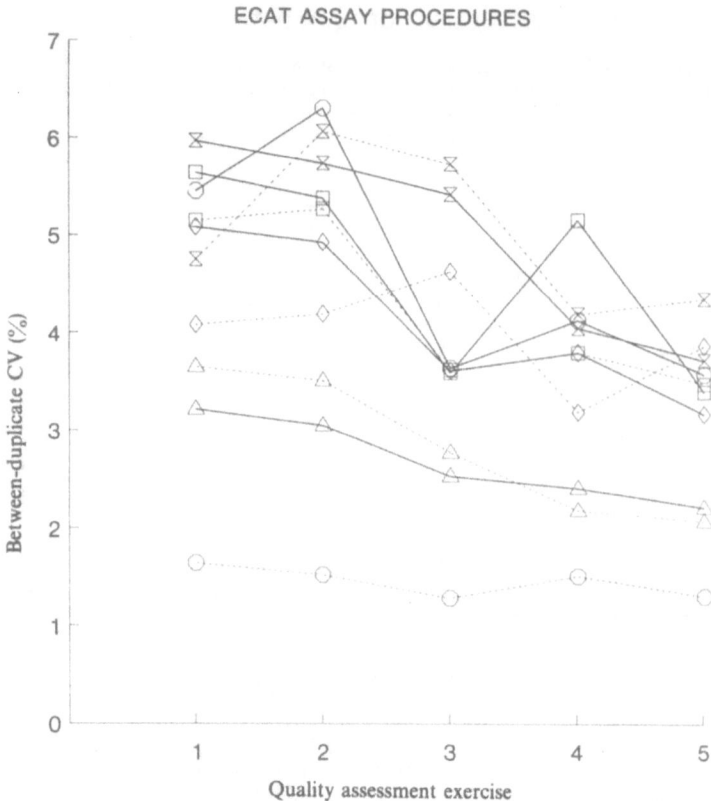

ECAT ASSAY PROCEDURES

Figure 1.4 Changes in between-duplicate CVs for 10 assays over five sequential QA exercises, averaged over 15 laboratories

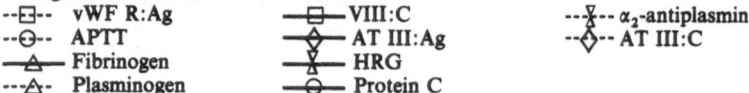

--□-- vWF R:Ag   --□-- VIII:C   --✕-- α₂-antiplasmin

--⊖-- APTT   --◇-- AT III:Ag   --◇-- AT III:C

--△-- Fibrinogen   --Ⴘ-- HRG

--△-- Plasminogen   --⊙-- Protein C

laboratories, the ultimate aim of any QA scheme, was of course disappointing, but this no doubt reflects more generally the difficulty in standardizing the performance of haemostatic tests.

DISCUSSION

The ECAT QA scheme, designed for monitoring performance in a particular multicentre study, differs from national QA schemes, such as the UK NEQAS in blood coagulation[3] and the College of American Pathologists' Surveys[4], which involve much larger numbers of participants from routine laboratories. The remit of the national schemes does not include internal QA, and so their assessment of performance is generally based on single results reported by each laboratory. This contrasts with ECAT QA scheme in which aspects of internal QA (between-duplicate and between-day variability) were explicitly

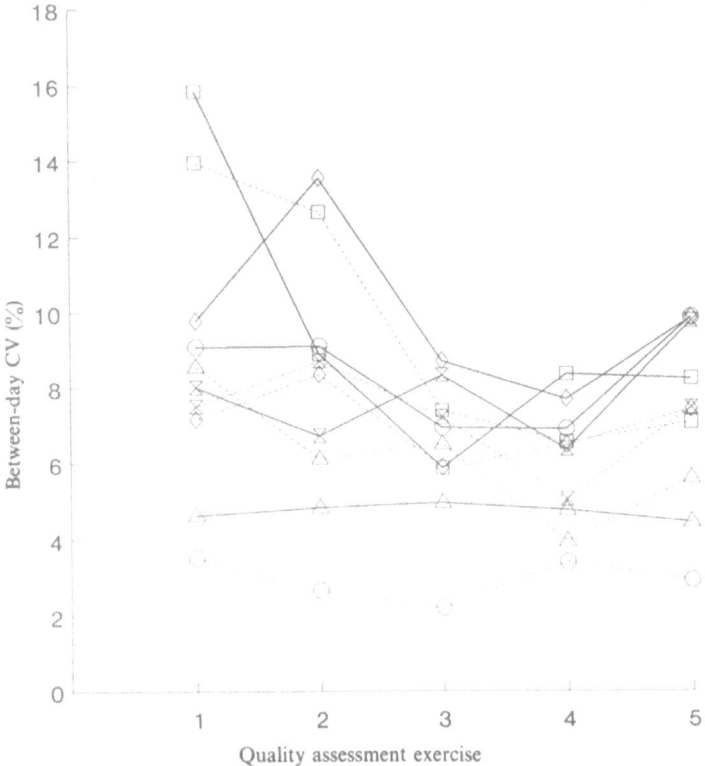

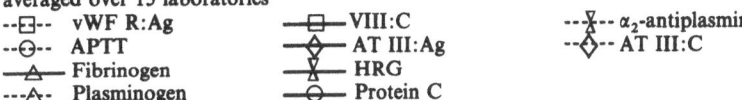

Figure 1.5 Changes in between-day CVs for 10 assays over five sequential QA exercises, averaged over 15 laboratories

--▣-- vWF R:Ag   ▬▣▬ VIII:C   --☒-- α_2-antiplasmin
--⊖-- APTT   ▬◇▬ AT III:Ag   --◇-- AT III:C
▬△▬ Fibrinogen   ▬☒▬ HRG
---△- Plasminogen   ▬⊖▬ Protein C

assessed to aid the speedy improvement of poor performance in individual laboratories.

Good performance in ECAT QA exercises of course does not guarantee good performance for the patients' samples in the main ECAT studies. Performance may be better for what are known to be QA samples, and aspects of blood sampling, handling and storage are not tested by such a scheme. However, it is certainly unlikely that a laboratory performing poorly in a QA exercise will perform adequately in the main study.

The possibility of analysing centrally all 3000 patients' samples in the first of the ECAT studies, the Angina Pectoris Study, proved impractical. In the more recent and somewhat smaller ECAT studies, the Deep Vein Thrombosis and Angioplasty studies, central analysis of the majority of the haemostatic tests is now considered feasible. However, similar QA schemes are continuing in these studies for the tests performed locally. Performance of analytical work locally in each laboratory stimulates a real collaboration between

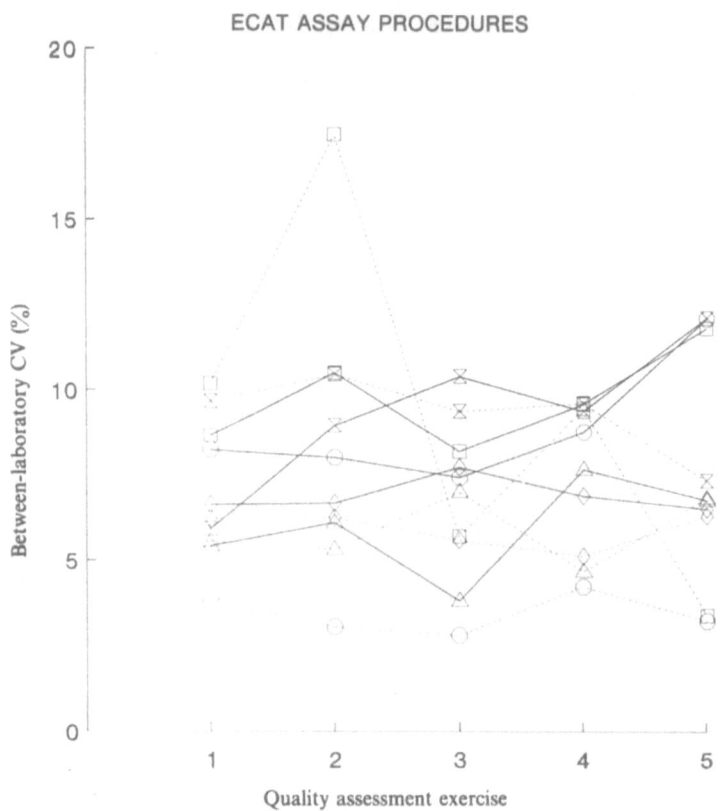

ECAT ASSAY PROCEDURES

Figure 1.6 Changes in between-laboratory CVs for 10 assays over five sequential QA exercises, averaged over 15 laboratories

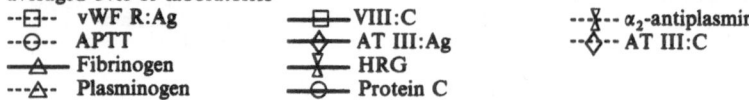

--⊟-- vWF R:Ag   —⊟— VIII:C   --⊠-- α_2-antiplasmin
--⊖-- APTT   —◆— AT III:Ag   --◇-- AT III:C
—△— Fibrinogen   —⊠— HRG
---△-- Plasminogen   —⊖— Protein C

centres, and means that the final results will be widely applicable because they have been obtained under typical laboratory conditions. In a multicentre study where patients' samples are to be assayed in different laboratories, a coordinated QA scheme is a prerequisite for success. However, such a scheme is useful in its own right in establishing awareness and critical assessment of each laboratory's performance in relation to that of others.

APPENDIX

For each assay, laboratory and QA exercise, three coefficients of variation (CVs) were calculated as follows:

1. Between-duplicate CV (based on single determinations within one analytical batch):

10

$$CV_1 = \sqrt{\sum_{i=1}^{10} (\log_e r_i)^2/20} \times 100\%$$

where the r_i are the ten ratios such as those shown in Figure 1.1.

2. Between-day CV (based on the means of duplicate determinations, on different days):

$$CV_2 = \sqrt{\sum_{i=1}^{5} (\log_e s_i)^2/10} \times 100\%$$

where the s_i are the five ratios such as those shown in Figure 1.2.

3. Between-laboratory CV (based on the means of four estimations, two duplicates on each of two days):

$$CV_3 = \sqrt{\sum_{i=1}^{5} (\log_e t_i - m_i)^2/4} \times 100\%$$

where the t_i are the five ratios such as those shown in Figure 1.3, and the m_i are the means of the $\log_e t_i$ for each sample, averaged over all the laboratories.

References

1. Report from the European Concerted Action on Thrombosis and Disabilities (ECAT). The measurement of haemostatic factors in 16 European laboratories: quality assessment for the mutlticentre ECAT Angina Pectoris Study. Thromb Haemostas 1989; 61: 301–6.
2. Report from the European Concerted Action on Thrombosis and Disabilities (ECAT). The impact of sequential quality assessment exercises on laboratory performance: the multicentre ECAT Angina Pectoris Study. Thromb Haemostas 1991; 65: 149–52.
3. Poller L. United Kingdom external quality assessment in blood coagulation: the first 21 years. J Clin Pathol 1989; 42: 1–3.
4. Triplett DA, Kopke JA. External quality control programs in coagulation testing: past, present and future. In: Triplett DA., ed. Advances in coagulation testing: interpretation and application. Skokie, IL: College of American Pathologists, 1985; 258–88.

2
Blood collection and preparation: pre-analytical variation

J. M. THOMSON

INTRODUCTION

The quality and success of the ECAT clinical studies, in particular the multicentre studies, largely depend on the method of blood collection, subsequent handling and plasma storage. The amount of care given to these aspects is ultimately reflected in the accuracy of the result. As soon as blood is withdrawn from a vessel, changes take place in the components of blood coagulation and haemostasis, e.g. platelet activation, release of tissue factor and initiation of clotting. In addition certain components become activated whereas others are labile and deteriorate. Observance of recommended criteria in the pre-analytical phase reduces the possibility of *in vitro* changes and contributes considerably towards the reliability of the test results. The aim is to achieve optimal preservation of the specimen in order that laboratory analyses reflect the *in vivo* state[1].

A protocol for blood collection and storage has been designed by the ECAT Assay Committee for these studies, to which all participants are requested to conform strictly. The various stages and recommendations have been presented during whole-day instruction courses held in Leiden, prior to commencement of the studies. Representatives from each centre, actively engaged in the project, i.e. technologists and clinicians, were invited to attend. Thus, opportunity was given to all centres to gain a full understanding of the study protocol and of a standardized method for the collection, preparation and storage of the blood specimens. These occasions also provided opportunity for discussion with the Project Leader and laboratory coordinators of any areas of misunderstanding of the protocol. The aim was to ensure that each centre was fully aware of the required criteria, at an early stage, prior to recruitment of patients. In addition participants from the various countries represented were able to meet one another and discuss the proposals informally.

Uniformity in pre-analytical variables is desirable in all coagulation laboratories and is particularly important in multicentre studies where plasmas from a number of centres are subjected to central analysis. In the ECAT studies the majority of the tests are carried out on frozen plasma by designated experts, following redistribution of the plasma samples from a central laboratory in Leiden.

COLLECTION, PREPARATION AND STORAGE OF BLOOD SAMPLES

The precise instructions provided in the ECAT study manuals for the collection and handling of blood samples for the DVT and PTCA studies are given in the appendices to this chapter. Some amplification and discussion of the details contained within them is given below.

Patient requirements prior to blood collection

The protocol stipulates that all blood specimens should be collected before 10 a.m. from patients who are resting and fasting. Some tests of coagulation, platelet function and fibrinolysis are known to be affected by food intake, particularly when containing fat. Likewise, stress and exercise can also have an effect; hence the necessity for the patient to be in a resting state. The influences of diet, stress and exercise on haemostasis have been well reviewed by Ogston[2]. The importance of a standard time of the day for blood coagulation is due to the influence of circadian rhythm. The fibrinolytic mechanism, for instance, shows a diurnal fluctuation with activity being lowest in the early morning and at a peak during the late afternoon[3].

Venipuncture technique

In order to standardize the blood collection procedure the ECAT Executive Committee have recommended since 1987 the use of Vacutainers (Becton Dickinson) for the DVT and PTCA studies, issued centrally to the participant laboratories. An essential prerequisite in any study of blood coagulation and fibrinolysis is the need for glass surfaces with which the blood will come into contact, to be well siliconized in order to reduce surface contact so that activation of clotting factors (e.g. F VII and F XII) and fibrinolytic parameters is minimized[4-6]. Citrated Vacutainers are claimed by their manufacturers to be well siliconized. The ECAT protocol advises that the tubes should be pre-cooled in a mixture of crushed ice and water prior to use in order to preserve those components which deteriorate more rapidly at higher temperatures.

Only minimal stasis should be applied to the upper arm prior to venipuncture. A good, clean entry to the vein is required, using a multisample needle (20 gauge), supplied with the Vacutainers. The patient's arm must be supported, in a downward position during this procedure and the tourniquet should be released as soon as blood enters the first collection tube. The tubes must be held steady until the vacuum is exhausted and blood flow ceases. Changing over to successive collection tubes should proceed quickly, avoiding any delay. Those containing an anticoagulant are mixed gently by inversion five times. Specifications for vacuum tubes and guidelines for their use have been published by National (USA) and European Committees for Clinical Laboratory Standards (NCCLS and ECCLS)[7-10]. The tubes should not be used beyond their expiration date. Maintenance of the vacuum is of utmost importance in obtaining constant citrate/blood ratios.

Anticoagulation of the blood

The anticoagulant in the Vacutainers provided for blood collection for coagulation and fibrinolytic parameters is buffered citrate, 3.2% (0.105 mol/L) containing citric acid. Concentrations ranging from 0.100 to 0.120 mol/L are acceptable according to ECCLS[9]. The NCCLS[11] recommended 0.109 or 0.129 mol/L. Addition of buffer is said to be effective in preserving the activity of certain clotting factors[12].

Blood samples in the PTCA study required for platelet factor 4 (PF4) and β-thromboglobulin (βTG) are collected into Vacutainers with an anticoagulant containing platelet release inhibitors. The mixture consists of citric acid, theophylline, adenosine and dipyridamole (CTAD). The latter is stated to inhibit platelet release, provided the tests are performed within 1 h of blood collection[13,14] (see also Chapter 3).

Following collection blood samples for coagulation and fibrinolysis are immediately transferred to a container of crushed ice and water. Those for blood chemistry and platelet count are maintained at room temperature.

Centrifugation

Blood collected into buffered citrate and into the anticoagulant containing platelet inhibitors (CTAD) must be centrifuged within 30 min of venipuncture. The time interval between collection of the sample, centrifugation and separation of the supernatant plasma may be crucial to the accuracy of the result. A speed of 2000g for 30 min is recommended in order to obtain plasma which is sufficiently platelet-poor. The temperature of the centrifuge is set at $+4\,^{\circ}$C.

Separation of the plasma, freezing and storage

Plasma is removed from the red cells immediately following centrifugation by carefully pipetting off, with a non-contact pipette, into a small plastic container of 25–50 ml capacity. Caution should be observed during this procedure to ensure that the platelet layer is not disturbed. This is particularly important with the CTAD samples, required for platelet function tests.

15

The pooled plasma is carefully mixed and aliquoted without delay into pre-cooled, well-identified containers which are supplied by ECAT to all participant centres. The volumes required for the various tests are specified in detail in Tables 2.1 and 2.2. Containers are firmly capped and snap-frozen immediately in order to maintain the quality of the sample. Altogether, 25 plasma aliquots are stored from each individual patient in both the DVT and PTCA studies. These include extras or 'back-up' samples which may be required for repeat testing or additional tests. Most of these samples are required for specific assays performed at single, expert centres. A small volume of the plasma is kept at room temperature for tests which are performed locally (see next section).

The method employed for snap-freezing of the plasma is very important in order to preserve the various plasma components to be measured. If liquid nitrogen is available this should be the method of choice. The process can also be achieved by the use of a refrigerated bath at $-50\,^{\circ}\mathrm{C}$ or a mixture of dry ice and acetone. Care must be taken, in this case, to ensure the containers are resistant to acetone. Those supplied for the project are suitable for this purpose; 2 ml tubes, with flat bottom and screw cap (Sarstedt). If none of these methods are locally available the plasma aliquots should be put into a deep-freeze at the lowest possible temperature available, to ensure rapid cooling and freezing. Once snap-frozen, long-term storage should be maintained

Table 2.1 ECAT DVT Study

Analysis	Volume for duplicate assays	
APTT	1×0.4 ml	
PT	1×0.4 ml	
Fibrinogen	1×0.4 ml	
Factor VII activity	1×0.4 ml	
Factor VIII activity	1×0.4 ml	
VWF antigen	1×0.4 ml	
AT III antigen	1×0.4 ml	
AT III activity	1×0.4 ml	
PC activity	1×0.4 ml	
PC antigen	1×0.4 ml	25×0.4 ml in sample storage box for central analysis
PS antigen	1×0.4 ml	
Alpha$_2$ AP activity	1×0.4 ml	
t-PA antigen	1×0.4 ml	
PAI antigen	1×0.4 ml	
PAI activity	1×0.4 ml	
FDP	1×0.4 ml	
HRGP antigen	1×0.4 ml	
Back-up samples	8×0.4 ml	
APTT	1×0.4 ml	
PT	1×0.4 ml	snap-frozen for local analysis
Fibrinogen	1×0.4 ml	
APTT	1×0.4 ml	
PT	1×0.4 ml	room temperature for local analysis (within 1 h of collection)
Fibrinogen	1×0.4 ml	

Table 2.2 ECAT PTCA Study

Analysis	Volume for duplicate assays	
β-Thromboglobulin	0.4 ml	
Platelet factor 4	0.4 ml	
Back-up CTAD-plasma	0.4 ml	
Fibrinogen	1×0.4 ml	
Factor VII activity	1×0.4 ml	
Factor VIII activity	1×0.4 ml	
VWF antigen	1×0.4 ml	
AT III antigen	1×0.4 ml	
AT III activity	1×0.4 ml	
PC antigen	1×0.4 ml	
PC activity	1×0.4 ml	25×0.4 ml in sample storage box for central analyses
PS antigen	1×0.4 ml	
Alpha$_2$ AP activity	1×0.4 ml	
t-PA antigen	1×0.4 ml	
PAI antigen	1×0.4 ml	
PAI activity	1×0.4 ml	
FDP	1×0.4 ml	
HRGP antigen	1×0.4 ml	
Back-up samples	7×0.4 ml	
APTT	0.4 ml	room temperature for local analysis (within 1 h of collection)

at a temperature below $-30\,°C$. Thawing and re-freezing of plasma is not permitted under any circumstances.

APPENDIX I: BLOOD SAMPLING AND HANDLING IN ECAT STUDIES

A. Sample collection

1. The blood samples are taken before 10 a.m. from patients who are resting and fasting (light breakfast without fat).
2. Only one technique of blood collection i.e. Vacutainers (Becton Dickinson) is allowed for the study.

Tubes required for blood collection are as follows:
DVT Study
one Vacutainer (plain), 5.0 ml for blood chemistry
four Vacutainers (citrate), 10.0 ml × 4 for coagulation and fibrinolytic tests, pre-cooled in crushed ice and water
one Vacutainer (EDTA), 4.0 ml for platelet count

PTCA Study
one Vacutainer (plain), 5.0 ml for blood chemistry
one Vacutainer (CTAD), 5.0 ml for platelet factors
three Vacutainers (citrate), 10.0 ml × 3 for coagulation and fibrinolytic tests
one Vacutainer (EDTA), for platelet and leucocyte count

17

3. Minimal stasis must be applied. There must be sufficient blood flow. A 20-gauge multi-sample needle (supplied) is used which should not be moved during withdrawal of blood from the vein.
4. If venipuncture is unsuccessful, or there is failure to collect sufficient blood from one arm, a further attempt should be made on the other arm.
5. The tubes are filled in the order indicated in (2), with minimum delay. All tubes must be completely filled. Citrated blood samples are gently mixed immediately after collection by inverting five times.
6. Tubes for blood chemistry and platelet count are maintained at room temperature. The five citrated tubes for coagulation and fibrinolysis are placed in crushed ice and water immediately following collection, for transit to the laboratory.

B. Centrifugation

Citrated blood is centrifuged as soon as possible and not later than 30 min after venipuncture. The minimal conditions are: $2000g$ for 30 minutes in a cold centrifuge with swing-out rotor (temperature setting $+4\,°C$).

C. Plasma separation

Carefully pipette off plasma into a small plastic container using a plastic (non-contact) pipette of 25–50 ml capacity. Mix gently and aliquot without delay into pre-cooled and well-identified tubes (Sarstedt), supplied and labelled for the project by ECAT, according to the scheme in Table 2.1 for the various coagulation and fibrinolytic tests. Pre-printed, dry fix labels (30×15 mm) containing the centre number, the patient's number and the name of the study are provided. In the PTCA study 1.5 ml of plasma should be carefully pipetted from the supernatant plasma in the CTAD tube *without disturbing the platelet layer* into a plastic tube. From this tube three pre-cooled and well-identified tubes will be filled for β-thromboglobulin (βTG), platelet factor 4 (PF4) and a back-up sample.

D. Freezing of plasma aliquots

All samples to be stored for assay at a later date must be snap frozen (see section E). This can be achieved with liquid nitrogen, a refrigerated bath at $-50\,°C$ or a mixture of dry ice and ethanol. If snap-freezing is not possible the tubes should be put in a deep-freeze at the lowest possible temperature, to ensure rapid cooling and freezing. Following snap-freezing, all of the plasma aliquots from a single patient are placed into a storage box containing 25 compartments (Nalgene, Nalge Company, Rochester, New York) supplied by ECAT for the study, and returned immediately into a freezer. Each box is labelled on the outside with the patient's number. Long-term storage should be maintained below $-30\,°C$ and preferably at $-70\,°C$. Thawing and re-freezing of plasma is not permitted. The total time between blood collection and plasma freezing should not exceed 90 min and should preferably be achieved in < 60 min.

E. General note

The only tests performed locally are the PT, APTT and fibrinogen. These are carried out twice. On the first occasion the tests are done on fresh plasma (stored at room temperature). They are repeated on deep-frozen samples (within 1 week).

APPENDIX II: AN EXAMPLE OF METHOD FOR TRANSPORT OF FROZEN SAMPLES

A system has been devised whereby frozen plasma samples, stored at the participant laboratories, are transported to the project leader. The following requirements are stipulated:

1. Stored plasmas are to be transported, in dry ice, in convenient batches. Sufficient dry ice must be obtained in order to keep the plasma frozen for at least 48 h (i.e. 10–12 kg).
2. Before organizing transport, the project leader must be contacted in advance. Parcels should be sent only on Tuesdays. This gives centres the opportunity to order sufficient dry ice and avoids transport during the weekend.
3. The carrier must provide a laboratory-to-laboratory service. The project leader makes clear arrangements in advance.
4. Parcels should be labelled 'URGENT', 'DRY ICE' and contain the address and telephone number of the project leader.
5. Samples from at least 20 patients should be sent in one transport, or from patients recruited over half a year.

References

1. Thomson JM. Specimen collection for blood coagulation testing. In: Koepke JA, ed., Laboratory haematology (2nd ed.). New York: Churchill Livingstone; 1991: 313.
2. Ogston D. ed., The physiology of hemostasis. London: Croom Helm; 1983: 267.
3. Cepelak R, Barcol H, Cepelakova H, Mayer, O. Circadian rhythm of fibrinolysis. In: Davidson JF, Rowan RM, Samama M, Desnoyers PC, eds., Progress in chemical fibrinolysis and thrombolysis, vol. 3. New York: Raven Press; 1978: 71.
4. Seligsohn U, Østerud B, Brown S et al. Activation of human factor VII in plasma and in purified systems. J Clin Invest 1979; 64: 1056.
5. Seligsohn U, Østerud B, Griffin JH, Rapaport SI. Evidence for the participation of both activated factor XII and activated factor IX in cold-promoted activation of factor VII. Thromb Res 1978; 13: 1049.
6. Iatridis SG, Ferguson JH. Effect of surface and Hageman factor on the endogenous or spontaneous activation of the fibrinolytic system. Thromb Diath Haemorrh 1961; 6: 411.
7. National Committee for Clinical Laboratory Standards. Procedures for the collection of diagnostic blood specimens by venipuncture. NCCLS document H3-A2 Villanova PA NCCLS; 1984.

8. European Committee for Clinical Laboratory Standards. Standard for specimen collection. Part 2: Blood specimen by Venipuncture, vol. 4, 1, 1987.
9. European Committee for Clinical Laboratory Standards. Standard for specimen collection. Part 1: Blood containers, vol. 3, 1, 1983.
10. National Committee for Clinical and Laboratory Standards. Evacuated tubes for blood specimen collection, 2nd ed. Approved standard H1-A2. NCCLS, Villanova PA, 1980.
11. National Committee for Clinical Standards. Collection, transport and preparation of blood specimens for coagulation testing and performance of coagulation assays: Approved guideline. NCCLS document H21-A, Villanova PA, 1986.
12. Godfrey R, Rhymes IL, Bidwell E, Barrowcliffe TW. The buffering of anticoagulants for blood coagulation. Thromb Diath Haemorrh 1975; 34: 879.
13. Contant G, Gouault-Heilmann M, Martinoli JL. Heparin inactivation during blood storage: Its prevention by blood collection in citric acid, theophylline, adenosine, dipyridamole–CTAD mixture. Thromb Res 1983; 31: 365.
14. Van den Besselaar AMHP, Meeuwisse-Braun J, Jansen-Gruter R, Bertina RM. Monitoring heparin therapy by the activated partial thromboplastin time – the effect of pre-analytical conditions. Thromb Haemostas 1987; 57: 226.

3
Beta-thromboglobulin and platelet factor 4

D. S. PEPPER and C. V. PROWSE

INTRODUCTION TO THE ASSAYS OF BETA-THROMBOGLOBULIN (BTG) AND PLATELET FACTOR 4 (PF4)

These two low molecular weight basic proteins are found almost exclusively in the alpha-granules of platelets and represent two of the earliest examples of the group of proteins now known collectively as the small inducible gene (SIG) family of proteins[1]. For a more detailed description of the early developments leading up to the development of these two assays the interested reader is referred to a recent review chapter[2].

Essentially, the specificity of the assay resides in the localization of the two marker proteins within the platelet granules and the sensitivity depends upon the large difference between their concentrations in platelets and plasma – thus even a small amount of platelet activation and release *in vivo* can lead to a measurable increase in the circulating levels of BTG and/or PF4. Of course such sensitivity also carries with it the need to avoid artifactual triggering of platelet release during the blood collection and separation processes. In this regard it has been found that problems in the BTG/PF4 assays can most often be ascribed to the blood sampling procedure rather than the assays themselves.

Physiological roles

Although BTG and PF4 are closely related in terms of structure[3], by contrast their functions are very different. PF4 has been known for many years as an inhibitor of heparin, and more recently has been shown to inhibit collagenase and angiogenesis, and to be chemotactic for several cell types. More recently, PF4 has been shown to reverse immunosuppression in certain animal models[4]. These various activities and the nomenclature of the various molecular forms are summarized in Table 3.1. BTG has less obvious biological

21

Table 3.1 Nomenclature and physiological properties of PF4 and βTG and related proteins

	PF4	PBP	LA PF4/CTAP III	βTG	NAP-2
pI (isoelectric point)	–	10	8	7	–
Amino acids per subunit	70	94	85	81	≥70
N-terminal residue	Glu	Ser	Asn	Ala	
Properties					
1. Heparin neutralization	++		+	±	
2. Endothelial binding	++			±	
3. Chemotactic for:					
Monocytes	++				
Neutrophils	±			±	?
Fibroblasts	±			±	
4. Inhibition contact activity	++		±		
5. Stimulates elastase	±		±		
6. Inhibits collagenase	++		–		
7. Inhibits megakaryocytopoiesis	++		+	±	
8. Inhibits angiogenesis	++		+		
9. Inhibition of bone resorption	±				
10. Mitogenic for:					
Fibroblasts		±	±	–	
Synovial cells		±	±	–	
3T3 cells		–	–	–	
11. Stimulates glycosaminoglycan synthesis			+		
12. Stimulates glucose uptake and lactate production			++		
13. Induces fibroblast plasminogen activator			++		
14. Enhances protacyclin production from endothelium					
15. Immunoregulatory effect	+		±	±	
16. Activates neutrophils					
Elastase release	±	–	–	–	++
Chemotaxis		–	–	–	++
Increases cell calcium		–	–	–	+

Table 3.1 (*Contd*)

Notes

1. All thromboglobulins derive from one gene and precursor protein.
2. See Kaplan KK, Niewiarowski S. Nomenclature of platelet proteins. Thromb Haemostas 1985, 53: 282–4 for a proposed standardized nomenclature of these proteins.
3. The pI8 form of thromboglobulin is the major form found in platelets.
4. The nomenclature of platelet granule proteins is unfortunately confusing.

PBP = Platelet basic protein with N-terminal sequence of: Ser-Ser-Thr-Lys-Gly-Gln-Thr-Lys-Arg-Asn-Leu-Ala-Lys-Gly-Lys-Glu ...

LAPF4/CTAPIII = Low affinity platelet factor 4/connective tissue activating protein III with N-terminal sequence of: Asn-Leu-Ala-Lys-Gly-Lys-Glu ...

βTG = Beta-thromboglobulin with N-terminal sequence of: Gly-Lys-Glu ...

Apart from these differences in the N-terminal sequence (due to progressive proteolytic cleavage) the sequences of all the proteins are identical.

functions but it can be deduced from its inclusion in the SIG family that it has a role to play in the various mechanisms of local inflammation and control[5], which follow on from activation of the haemostatic mechanisms and precede tissue remodelling. A degradation product of BTG, neutrophil activating peptide 2, has a role in the activation and chemotaxis of neutrophils.

Pathophysiological role

Very little is known about the role of the platelet proteins BTG and PF4 in pathophysiology, although the co-secreted platelet-derived growth factor does appear to stimulate fibrosis and possibly atherosclerosis. The strong binding of PF4 to glycosaminoglycans which are present on the endothelial lining of blood vessels means that local activation and release of platelet PF4 can change the endothelial cell surface from a weakly anticoagulant surface into a potentially procoagulant one. Likewise, local activation and release within the kidneys can neutralize the cell surface charge and hence the selective permeability of the kidneys to macro-molecules. PF4 has been found in high concentrations within perivascular mast cells associated with sprouting capillaries in inflamed and regenerating tissues, but it is not known if this is cause or effect[6].

The BTG family of proteins (modified by sequential proteolysis *in vivo* at both N and C termini) have been implicated in stimulation of a variety of cell types to undergo proliferation which may well be part of the tissue remodelling process subsequent upon inflammation and damage (Table 3.1).

METHODS OF ASSAY

Principles and assay characteristics

During the period of the ECAT studies, a choice of 'home-made'[7] and commercial assays has been available in both RIA and ELISA formats. In view of the advantages of uniform assay methods, reagents and strict quality control it was recommended that all participants used the commercial RIA kits for BTG (Amersham) and PF4 (Abbott), and if this was not possible then the commercial ELISAs (BTG and PF4 from Stago or PF4 from Behring). Because the latter were available only towards the end of the project the majority of workers have used the commercial RIA kits.

A series of training courses was organized in Edinburgh to provide training for operators in both blood sampling and assay operations. It soon became clear that the majority of the problems arose in the blood sampling and processing, whereas in contrast the assay kits themselves were remarkably trouble-free. For this reason we shall stress in this chapter the sampling procedure rather more than the assays themselves. Fortunately, once platelet-free plasma has been correctly obtained, the BTG and PF4 antigens are remarkably stable under the usual conditions of storage of plasma.

As with many other RIAs the assay principles are based on the use of a limited amount of high-affinity antibody binding a significant proportion of a ^{125}I labelled pure protein (antigen) tracer. In the presence of sample antigen the proportion of bound tracer is reduced and the amount of bound tracer is quantitated by gamma counting after precipitation of bound antigen.

The ELISA assays are also of the common 'sandwich' format using two antibodies – one immobilized on a plastic microtitre plate or tube and the other conjugated to an enzyme. The 'sandwich' is held together with the antigen in the middle. Unlike RIAs, with these ELISAs the increasing amount of antigen is followed by an increasing strength of signal, which is the exact opposite of RIAs. As with all immunoassays the range is limited to a factor of about 10-fold so any high values must be diluted in an appropriate diluent to be within range.

Low values are more problematic, but in the case of urine BTG it may be feasible to modify the kits for BTG by delayed addition of tracer to diluted antibody and extended incubation so as to improve the sensitivity[8].

Venipuncture and sample handling

This aspect of the assays deserves great attention to detail – more than is usually given. For instance, it is worthwhile to train the blood taking and processing staff specifically rather than simply delegating the job to routine nursing or clinical staff. It cannot be overstressed that the quality of BTG and PF4 assays starts at the bedside with careful blood sampling!

A number of techniques are possible and can be ranked in terms of desirability. These are: (1) simple syringe and needle, (2) Vacutainer and needle, (3) butterfly cannula and syringe, (4) indwelling cannula. Generally, the less trauma used (including tourniquet), and the quicker the sample is taken, the better. If possible avoid excessive negative pressure on the syringe and do not use the first few drops of blood to emerge. Indwelling catheters should be used as soon as possible after insertion and certainly not more than 45 min after insertion. Cooling of syringes, collection tubes and anticoagulant before sampling is desirable and after sampling is essential. We recommend chipped ice (flaked ice, not cubes) which is moistened with saline so as to improve thermal contact but not so much as to make it fluid, as then the empty tubes may fall over.

For convenience in standardizing techniques across many European countries it was felt desirable to use a system that was commercially available, stable and acceptable to the majority of centres. For these reasons the Becton Dickinson CTAD Vacutainer system was chosen as the recommended common anticoagulant. However, as shown in Table 3.2, a number of other anticoagulants can be used, and with care will give comparable results.

Anticoagulants

The various types of anticoagulants used are summarized in Table 3.2. There are advantages and disadvantages to each of these. The ETP (Edinburgh)

ECAT ASSAY PROCEDURES

Table 3.2 Anticoagulants used for βTG/PF4 assays

Composition	ETP (local)	Becton Dickinson CTAD-Vacutainer and Diatube-H (Stago)	Thrombotect (Abbott)	ET Amersham*
EDTA	78 mmol/L	–	2.5% = 67 mmol/L	78 mmol/L
Citrate	–	109 mmol/L	–	–
Theophylline	10 mmol/L	15 mmol/L	–	10 mmol/L
Prostaglandin E_1	0.33 µg/ml	–	–	–
Adenosine	–	3.7 mmol/L	–	–
Dipyridamole	–	0.2 mmol/L	–	–
Procaine HCl	–	–	7% = 258 mmol/L	–
2-Chloroadenosine	–	–	0.02% = 0.83 mmol/L	–
Tube	Local glass	Glass Vacutainer	Glass Vacutainer	Plastic
Ratio blood/anticoagulant	9:1	9:1	9:1	9:1
Blood (ml) added to ml anticoagulant	2.7 to 0.3	4.5 to 0.5	4.5 to 0.5	2.7 to 0.3

Due to the instability of PGE_1, ETP must be stored frozen.

*Lack of PGE_1 means blood samples must be processed to plasma within 5 h. Plastic tubes give poorer cooling than glass.

anticoagulant has to be home-made as it is not commercially available. It contains PGE_1, and therefore has to be kept frozen at $-40\,°C$ before use. The use of EDTA requires strict attention to cooling at or below $4\,°C$ throughout the separation process. The Amersham kit contains ET anticoagulant (i.e. Edinburgh cocktail without PGE_1) in plastic tubes, it is commercially available (and 'free' with each kit) and also has the advantage of being stable at room temperature; however, the plastic tubes do not cool as rapidly as glass, and the absence of PGE_1 tends to give higher normal values for BTG/PF4. The Abbott 'Thrombotect' anticoagulant is available commercially, separately from the PF4 assay kits. The Becton Dickinson CTAD (and Stago Diatube H) are both commercially available in the popular Vacutainer format, and the anticoagulant mixture is stable at room temperature and is not critically dependent on careful cooling to be useful, thus this anticoagulant is the one recommended for use by ECAT in the PTCA study.

Blood must be kept cold on ice and centrifuged within 3 h of collection. Sets of labelled tubes in sufficient numbers (ideally pairs) are placed in a swinging-bucket refrigerated centrifuge. This should have been pre-cooled and calibrated to guarantee that the samples will be centrifuged at $+2$ to $+4\,°C$ during spinning. If no accurate temperature monitoring is possible, use crystals or flakes of ice added to the bucket or placed on top of the tube cap(s). After running for the desired time/speed/temperature the ice crystals should still remain, but be careful not to undercool the centrifuge below $-1\,°C$ as the plasma may supercool and freeze when separating. The centrifuge should be capable of generating at least $1000g$ and should provide adequate support and cushioning for the tubes so that they do not break at speed. Generally, a $1000g$ spin for 45 min at $+2\,°C$ will provide adequate separation of platelets from plasma. Higher g forces and shorter run times are desirable if the tubes are strong enough to survive reliably. Where a refrigerated centrifuge is not available it may be feasible to use finely crushed ice (not cubes) surrounding each tube, for example a 100 ml bucket with 90 ml of crushed ice and one sample tube, i.e. four samples per rotor. It is not feasible to use a larger number of tubes per bucket because less ice is available and will melt in less than 30 min of centrifugation.

Following centrifugation the tubes should be allowed to decelerate gently without braking, particularly during the last $100-200$ rpm when remixing is most likely. The tubes should be very gently removed from the rotor and placed carefully and firmly in a rack that will not permit shaking, rattling or other sudden movements. From this point on no cooling is necessary provided plasma is separated within 5 min of the end of centrifugation.

Plasma should be separated very carefully as follows – if a 9 ml sample of blood was used then an automatic pipette set to 2 ml is used with a disposable polypropylene tip. The pipette tip is very gently passed through the meniscus layer and into the central third of the plasma without disturbing either the meniscus layer (often fatty) or the buffy coat; plasma is slowly and gently aspirated. The pipette is then slowly withdrawn and the 2 ml sample can be transferred to one, or preferably two, aliquot tubes pre-labelled with the patient's details. The samples can be assayed for both BTG and PF4, or one assay can be performed and the other done retrospectively on 'interesting' stored aliquots. Such separated samples for BTG/PF4 assays are quite stable and can be stored at 20°C for 24 h, at 4°C for 7 days and at −20°C for several years. If samples have to be shipped any distance by mail it is possible to add 1–2 µl of 20% w/v sodium azide to 0.7–1.4 ml of plasma and ship as a liquid in tightly stoppered tubes. The best tubes are Nunc (or similar) cryotubes with external threads and a silicone rubber 'O' ring, these obviate the risk of leakage which often occurs during air mail transport.

RIA kits

Assay procedures are well described by the manufacturers and enclosed in the kit. The two commercially available RIA kits are from Amersham for BTG and Abbott for PF4. The former gives 48 determinations (duplicates on five standards and 19 unknowns) in the range of 10–225 ng/ml and is completed in less than 2 h. The latter gives 100 determinations (duplicates on five standards and 43 unknowns) in the range 10–100 ng/ml in less than 3 h.

The manufacturers' kit literature is very comprehensive and has been used successfully in training many laboratory technicians from all the European countries. In our experience no problems are encountered in using these commercial kits, and we recommend their use. Additionally, the manufacturers' kit literature is copyright so we do not propose to reproduce it here.

The Amersham kit comes complete with a set of anticoagulant (ET) and tubes, as well as a useful polystyrene foam base and rack which serves as both a test-tube rack and ice-water container. The Abbott anticoagulant 'Thrombotect' is not supplied with the kit and has to be bought separately.

The Amersham kit may be modified by greater dilution and longer incubation periods to increase the sensitivity for screening of BTG in urine; however, this is at the expense of precision so the assay is more of a ± type, with a cut-off[8] around 0.4 ± 0.2 ng/ml.

Several general points can be made which apply to both kits. The method of separating 'bound' from 'free' counts is by ammonium sulphate precipitation of antibody-bound counts. Since the precision of this method depends on the total protein content of the samples, it is designed to be accurate with undiluted plasma samples. If samples are so high as to be off-scale (> 225 ng/ml for BTG and PF4 > 100 ng/ml; a situation which is rare in clinical practice and should itself give rise to suspicion) then any dilution must be made in a fluid such as horse serum or turkey serum which contains no crossreacting antigens and provides a similar protein milieu.

The assay standard curves are very steep at the low end and very shallow at the high end, which reduces accuracy at the extreme ends of the range. Greatest accuracy is achieved if sample values fall within the middle one-third of the standard curve. The manufacturers both arrange that this coincides with the upper end of the normal range, i.e. the cut-off between normal and pathological samples. The Abbott kit uses buffer as a zero standard; however, values below 10 ng/ml are likely to be inaccurate as this is not a true control so such values are best reported as < 10 ng/ml.

ELISA kits

Two manufacturers (Stago and Behring) offer commercial kits for PF4 and Stago offer a BTG kit as well as an anticoagulant. The various kits and details are summarized in Table 3.3. As they appeared later than the commercial RIAs there has been less experience with them, but we expect this situation to change as more people switch away from radioisotopes to ELISA. In our limited experience of these kits, they are quite adequate for the purposes of clinical screening. The kit insert leaflets give great detail for the operators and, as stated with RIA kits earlier, we do not intend to repeat the instructions here, for the same reasons. Several points can be mentioned, however, about these kits. The Stago kits do not provide an anticoagulant. Stago sell separately an anticoagulant mixture under the trade name 'Diatube H'. The Behring 'Enzygnost PF4' kit does include an anticoagulant but it is referred to as 'sampling medium' and is of undisclosed composition. In our experience any of the established anticoagulants can be used with any assay kit, whether RIA or ELISA.

The Stago kits use 96-well microtitre tray format whereas the Behring kit uses individual coated tubes.

The assay ranges are: Stago BTG 5–200 i.u./ml; Stago PF4 2.5–100 i.u./ml and Behring PF4 2–60 ng/ml. The Stago kit requires predilution of plasma samples (1:10 for BTG and 1:5 for PF4). Additionally, urine can be assayed for BTG at >0.2 i.u./ml if the urine sample is diluted only 1:2 (one international unit is approximately the same as 1 ng/ml – see later). Correlation with the RIA kits is claimed to be 0.95 by the ELISA kit manufacturers, and this is confirmed in our experience.

Evaluation of results, normal ranges, and source of error

Generally, we find no problems with the evaluation of results from commercial kit calibration curves. Provided careful pipetting and separating steps are used the individual duplicates should agree closely.

If the duplicates do not agree well one could take the mean result, but it is preferable to discard the values and repeat the assay. If values are below the lowest standards they should be reported as such. Urine values for BTG (but not PF4) can be reported as $\pm$ in modified versions of the Amersham RIA(8) and Stago ELISA. If high (see later) values are obtained, repeat the assays on the remaining duplicate frozen sample after dilution in animal plasma or serum. If high values are still obtained, it is recommended to obtain a fresh blood sample from the patient to rule out artifactual activation and release during venipuncture and blood processing. Since blood levels of BTG and PF4 can rise and fall over a matter of a day or so, it is worth re-sampling as soon as possible after a single high value is obtained. For studies involving serial sampling a pre-sample should be obtained to establish a baseline prior to any planned medical or surgical procedures, with daily sampling planned over a period of say 5 days around the procedure.

Table 3.3 Assay format

	Edinburgh	Amersham	Abbott	Stago	Behringwerke
Assay	BTG/PF4	BTG	PF4	Asserachrom BTG/PF4	PF4 'Enzygnost'
Format	Competitive RIA	Competitive RIA	Competitive RIA	Sandwich ELISA	Sandwich ELISA
Comment	Second antibody to separate complexes	Ammonium sulphate to separate complexes	Ammonium sulphate to separate complexes	Two-step	Two-step
Time	18–24h	2 or 6 h	3 h	2.5h	2.5 to 4.5h

30

Normal ranges

An essential part of setting up an assay is to establish the local normal range. This could be in students, laboratory staff, blood donors or better in patients; furthermore the patients should ideally cover the complete age range with e.g. $n = 10$ patients in each of the age spans 20–30, 30–40, 40–50, 50–60 and 60–70 years. The latter is sometimes difficult to achieve, but it is worth trying because BTG/PF4 levels tend to rise with increasing age. In Edinburgh the normal ranges for BTG were 20–50 ng/ml and for PF4 5–25 ng/ml (see Table 3.4). Other laboratories may find other values because of the combination of different patient populations, different blood sampling techniques, anticoagulants, assays and standards. In an attempt to simplify the problem of comparing numerical values between different laboratories, WHO international standards are now available for BTG and PF4 (see later). However, it is important to stress that from a clinical point of view the absolute numerical value is not as important as the value relative to the local normal range and cut-off. Whenever local staff or techniques are changed, the normal range should be re-established.

Sources of error

Sources of error are most often caused by blood sampling techniques or separation errors. Trained, skilled operators are the best insurance against these problems. Attention to detail in the venipuncture, cooling, centrifugation and separation step have already been mentioned as important. Once separated, the sample antigens are quite stable. It is quite unusual to find BTG and PF4 values above assay highest standards in any clinical situation.

Table 3.4 Normal levels

	BTG	PF4
Human		
Plasma (% serum)	37 ± 11 (0.20%)	14.7 ± 10 (0.10%)
Serum	18,000 ± 3650	14,800 ± 3400
Platelet	56 ± 1.2	64 ± 4.5
Whole blood	10,900 ± 1860	10,890 ± 2470
Urine (% plasma)	0.14 ± 0.009 (0.4%)	0.43 ± 0.2 (2.9%)
Amniotic fluid*	49 ± 35	5.6 ± 6.1
Synovial fluid*	57 ± 20	8.8 ± 6.2
Cerebrospinal fluid*	1.1 ± 0.5	<0.5
Saliva	0.3 ± 0.2	–
Baboon†		
Plasma (% serum)	5.2 ± 1.1 (0.14%)	3.2 ± 1.8 (0.12%)
Serum	3,755 ± 960	2,660 ± 1,135
Platelet	7.3 ± 2.0	5.0 ± 1.3

Values are in ng/ml, except platelet content is ng/10^6 cells.

* Some of these samples were from patients.

† From Bowen Pope DF et al. (Blood 1984; 64: 458) who used commercial RIA kits rather than the 'Edinburgh' assay format.

In the case of PF4 the prior administration of intravenous heparin can 'flush out' surface-bound PF4 from a pool sequestered on the vascular endothelium. Check for heparin administration within 90 min before sampling when high values are obtained. Chronic (subcutaneous) heparin does not elevate PF4 values after the first 6 h of treatment.

In the past it has been recommended that the ratio of PF4 to BTG can be used to discern if a blood sample has been correctly taken. Since in a normal person the ratio is 1:2 or 1:3 any deviation from this ratio (e.g. 1:1) is suspicious[9]. Unfortunately this rule does not apply in pathological situations in patients, so the method cannot be recommended where any disease process is operating. The mechanisms of clearance (and half-lives) of the two markers are quite different and so disease (e.g. in kidneys or liver) can differentially affect the clearance of BTG or PF4 without affecting the clearance of the other analyte. Where it is not feasible to measure both analytes we recommend studying BTG – because BTG assays are more sensitive and accurate and this analyte is not affected by heparin administration.

Where abnormally low platelet proteins are found it is wise to perform a platelet count, and where abnormally high platelet proteins are found this is also recommended, since BTG/PF4 levels tend to be influenced slightly by the platelet count. However, within the normal range of platelet count $(200–400 \times 10/L)$ there is no significant influence of platelet count on BTG or PF4.

Because RIAs and ELISAs are antibody-based they cannot generally be used in species other than humans. Limited crossreactivity does occur with primates and a few other species. The interested reader is referred to an earlier publication[10].

Heparin addition *in vitro* to samples, e.g. as an anticoagulant, will also raise PF4 levels by displacement from cell surfaces, tube surfaces, etc. This effect is much less dramatic than that seen following *in vivo* heparin administration. Catheters, especially those that have been indwelling for more than 45 min, can give erratic high values of BTG and PF4 and are best avoided. Likewise any invasive procedure such as extracorporeal circulation (heart–lung bypass, renal dialysis) and even blood transfusion with cellular components will raise BTG/PF4 for several hours after treatment. Indwelling prosthetic devices such as cardiac valves will also chronically raise BTG/PF4 levels.

In general if PF4:BTG ratio is 1:2 and both values are elevated then a genuine *in vivo* activation/release can be deduced. If BTG values are elevated, but PF4 is normal, suspect incipient kidney failure, with or without associated hypertension. Elevated PF4 values with normal BTG are commonly caused by heparin administration. Serial studies of PF4:BTG ratio in a single individual may be of more value than a single pair of values on one occasion.

Clinical interpretation

Interpretation of genuinely elevated BTG/PF4 values is still problematic in terms of clinical consequences. What we can say at this time is that BTG/PF4 assays are very useful to detect platelet activation and release *in vivo*. However, it remains to be seen how platelet release, as detected by BTG/PF4, may be of predictive value in any particular disease state. A large number of positive (and negative) correlations have been reported in the world literature and those up to 1986 have been summarized[2]. Unfortunately, although significant differences have repeatedly been shown between patient and normal *groups*, the scatter of values and overlap between normal and pathological ranges does not allow an unequivocal diagnosis from values obtained on a single occasion with a *single patient*.

STANDARDIZATION AND QUALITY CONTROL

In the early studies with BTG and PF4 assays (1975–85) individual users and manufacturers prepared their own standards. Inevitably variations occurred and 'normal' ranges reported for BTG varied by about 2-fold and PF4 by about 4-fold. In an attempt to regularize this situation the WHO standards for BTG and PF4 were produced by the National Institute for Biological Standards and Control (NIBSAC) in London. These purified standards[11] are designated as 83/501 for BTG and 83/505 for PF4. The vials contain respectively 500 i.u. (488 ng) and 400 i.u. (382 ng). However, it is important to stress that individual laboratories and assays will give different 'conversion factors', e.g. in Edinburgh the ratios are 1.63 (ng BTG/i.u.) and 1.69 (ng PF4/i.u.) so that results should be expressed in international units (i.u.). WHO reference vials are available from NIBSAC and can be used to calibrate local standards.

Quality control samples have been prepared in 2.0 ml freeze-dried ampoules by the authors, and distributed widely to ECAT participants. These have been chosen to fall on the borderline between normal and pathological ranges, i.e. approximately 60 ng/ml BTG and 30 ng/ml PF4. These ampoules are still available on application by interested participants. Ideally, such QC material should be included in every batch of assays run, and consistent values should be obtained. Generally, the RIAs and ELISAs do give consistent values and we believe this can be ascribed to the remarkable stability of BTG and PF4 antigens once they are properly prepared, combined with the careful quality control which is an intrinsic part of the manufacture of commercial kits.

References

1. St Charles R, Walz DA, Edwards BFP. The three dimensional structure of bovine platelet factor 4 at 3 Å resolution. J Biol Chem 1989; 264: 2092–9.
2. Pepper DS. Radioimmunoassay of platelet proteins. In: Patrono C, Pesker BA, eds., Handbook of experimental pharmacology, vol. 82. Berlin: Springer-Verlag, 1987; 517–41.
3. Walz DA. Platelet release proteins as molecular markers for the activation process. Sem. Thromb Hemostas 1984; 16: 270–9.
4. Gregg EO, Yarwood L, Wagstaffe MJ, Pepper DS, McDonald M. Immunomodulatory properties of platelet factor 4: prevention of concanavalin A suppressor induction in vitro and augmentation of an antigen specific delayed type hypersensitivity response *in vivo*. Immunology 1990; 70: 230–4.

5. Walz A, Dewald B, Tscharner W, Baggiolini M. Effects of the neutrophil activating peptide NAP-2, platelet basic protein, connective tissue activating peptide III and platelet factor 4 on human neutrophils. J Exp Med 1989; 170: 1745–50.
6. McClaren KM, Holloway L, Pepper DS. Human platelet factor 4 and tissue mast cells, Thromb Res 1980; 19: 293–7.
7. Bolton AE, Ludlam CA, Moore S, Pepper DS, Cash JD. Three approaches to the radioimmunoassay of human β-thromboglobulin. Br J Haematol 1976; 33: 233–8.
8. Van Oost BA, Veldhyzen B, Timmermans APM, Sixma JJ. Increased urinary β-thromboglobulin excretion in diabetes assayed with a modified RIA kit-technique. Thromb Haemostas 1983; 49: 18–20.
9. Arocha-Pinango CL, Ojeda A, Lopez G, Garcia L, Linares J. Beta-thromboglobulin (beta-TG) and Platelet Factor 4 (PF4) in obstetrical cases. Acta Obstet. Sci. 1985; 2: 115–20.
10. Dawes J, Clemetson KJ, Gogstad GO, McGregor J, Clezardin P, Prowse CV, Pepper DS. A radioimmunoassay for thrombospondin used in a comparative study of thrombospondin, β-thromboglobulin and platelet factor 4 in healthy volunteers. Thromb Res 1983; 29: 569–81.
11. Kerry PJ, Curtis AD. Standardization of β-thromboglobulin (βTG) and platelet factor 4 (PF4): a collaborative study to establish international standards for βTG and PF4. Thromb Haemostas 1985; 53: 51–5.

4
The activated partial thromboplastin time (APTT)

L. POLLER and J. M. THOMSON

The partial thromboplastin time is a global test for detection of abnormalities of 'intrinsic' clotting. The presence of an activator in the test system, to accelerate the test by effecting maximum activation, has led to it being referred to as the activated partial thromboplastin time (APTT). As well as shortening the test, the presence of an activator has increased the precision and reproducibility of the results by eliminating the variable effects of contact with glass surfaces previously encountered with non-activated PTT methods.

APTT PHOSPHOLIPIDS

The term partial thromboplastin is used to distinguish it from the complete thromboplastin of the prothrombin time test, since the APTT reagent lacks the apoprotein component of tissue thromboplastin. Partial thromboplastin consists of the phospholipid part of thromboplastin and is prepared from animal tissue or from vegetable sources. The phospholipid acts as a platelet substitute in the intrinsic system. The lipid composition of different APTT reagents, however, varies considerably. The total concentrations of phospholipid and fatty acid in some widely used APTT reagents have been shown to differ by as much as 300 times[1]. These discrepancies markedly affect responses to coagulation defects and inhibitors of coagulation. The requirements for the phospholipid component of the test system may also vary according to the nature of the clotting defect being measured. For example, the concentration of negatively charged phospholipids, e.g. phosphatidyl serine, has been shown to be critical[2].

OTHER COMPONENTS OF THE APTT TEST

Those which affect the clotting response include the type of activator, length of incubation with the plasma and the presence of buffers[3,4]. Particulate activators include kaolin, celite and micronized silica, whereas one commonly used activator, ellagic acid, is non-particulate. The amount of activator present in the various commercial techniques, and the length of incubation time employed with the plasma, show considerable variation. The effectiveness of an activator in the APTT is governed by many considerations, e.g. its concentration, the incubation time and the composition of the phospholipid. It is the combination of the activator with other components which appears to determine the reliability of the test[5]. The use of different types of coagulometer can also have a considerable effect on the clotting time[6].

SENSITIVITY OF THE APTT

A reliable APTT reagent should be sufficiently sensitive to record an abnormal result when the level of any single or combined intrinsic clotting factor deficiency is reduced to a level which may cause spontaneous bleeding, or haemorrhage following a haemostatic challenge. Proctor and Rapaport[7] stated that the APTT should be able to detect factor deficiencies of 30% or less. It should also be sufficiently sensitive to low concentrations of heparin whilst giving a linear response to graded concentrations of heparin, spanning a clinically relevant range.

CLINICAL USES

The main use of the APTT is for the screening of coagulation defects and the presence of inhibitors. The test is prolonged by deficiencies of factors VIII, IX, X, XI and XII and defects of the contact phase, e.g. prekallikrein, high molecular weight kininogen. It also may be prolonged by gross defects of factors II, V and fibrinogen. With a good APTT system specific and non-specific inhibitors of intrinsic clotting factors are detected. The degree of abnormality depends upon the responsiveness of a particular APTT method to a specific defect. When used as a screening test for lupus anticoagulants (LA) the detection rate is greatly influenced by the concentration and type of phospholipid content of the reagent. Reagents containing the highest concentrations of phospholipid tend to be less responsive to LA. The APTT is also the most widely used method for the laboratory monitoring of heparin administration[8,9]. Although other more specific techniques have been advocated, e.g. anti-Xa assays, the APTT has been almost universally preferred as it is regarded as a global test of coagulation which assesses the overall effect of heparin on clotting.

NEED FOR STANDARDIZATION

Because APTT results are influenced by changes in various different stages of the coagulation mechanism they are subject to more variables than specific clotting assays. The need for standardization of the APTT has been demonstrated in many reports, particularly with regard to the widespread application of the test in laboratory monitoring of heparin administration[3,10-15]. Possible methods of standardization are currently being evaluated in an international collaborative study under the joint auspices of the International Society for Haemostasis and Thrombosis and the International Committee for Standardization in Haematology.

PATHOPHYSIOLOGICAL VARIATION IN THE APTT

Stress, exercise, pregnancy, the post-partum state and surgical operations result in acceleration of the test. Prothrombotic changes associated with recent deep vein thrombosis, thromboembolic disorders and oestrogen administration may result in accelerated clotting times[4]. Acquired pathological states such as liver disease, DIC, and drug toxicity cause prolongation. Certain drugs, including oral anticoagulants, heparin and thrombolytic agents, prolong the APTT. The test is also prolonged in the newborn[16].

THE APTT IN THE EUROPEAN CONCERTED ACTION ON THROMBOSIS (ECAT) STUDIES

A single APTT reagent and technique was selected by the executive committee to be employed at all participant centres in the ECAT studies because of the variability of performance of the different APTT methods summarized earlier in this chapter, due to lack of standardization. The Manchester APTT was chosen as it has been shown in a number of published studies to give good sensitivity to a wide range of coagulation disorders and inhibitors[15]. The manual technique was selected for the ECAT studies because automated techniques may have marked and variable coagulometer effects on APTT results. To gain familiarity with the method, and to reduce the influence of interlaboratory variation in technique, representatives from all participant centres attended training courses organized by ECAT in Leiden. On-going programmes of external quality control have been conducted subsequently to monitor their performance (see Chapter 1).

THE MANCHESTER APTT METHOD

The reagent is a phospholipid extract of rabbit brain tissue which is prepared in lyophilized form for long-term stability. It is reconstituted with a physiological buffer (Owren's buffer, pH 7.35). The activator is light kaolin. Optimum sensitivity is achieved with an activation time of 10 min.

Details of technique

1. Lyophilized APTT reagent (store at −20 °C). Reconstitute by adding exactly 10 ml of cold Owren's buffer (see item 2, below). The stopper is replaced and it is mixed gently to resuspend. The diluted suspension is dispensed into small volumes, e.g. 1.0 ml amounts, using non-wettable containers which are tightly capped and immediately frozen (−20 °C to −40 °C). This procedure should be accomplished with minimum delay, preferably within 15 min from reconstitution. The frozen aliquots of the reagent are stable for at least 3 months.

   An aliquot of the diluted suspension should be thawed out rapidly when required by placing in a water bath at 37 °C for 1–2 min immediately before use. This is maintained in crushed ice prior to use. The reagent is stable for at least 2 h under these conditions. Any remaining reagent is discarded after use and it is not refrozen.
2. Owren's buffer (Sodium diethylbarbiturate (11.75 g) and sodium chloride (14.67 g) dissolved in 1570 ml distilled water and 430 ml 0.1 N hydrochloric acid, pH 7.35) for reconstitution of APTT reagent (store at +2 to 8 °C).
3. Light kaolin (0.25 g/100 ml) is suspended in Owren's buffer (store at +2 to 8 °C). It is mixed well before use. An aliquot is decanted when required into a separate container and any remainder is discarded.

Method

Testing should be performed on fresh plasma, collected and stored as indicated in Chapter 2, as soon as possible after collection and no longer than 1 h after venipuncture. The test plasma is kept in a stoppered polystyrene container at room temperature.

The kaolin suspension and calcium chloride are warmed in separate test tubes in a water bath at 37 °C. The following reagents are added in the order indicated without delay into a glass tube, pre-warmed in a water bath:

0.1 ml test plasma
0.1 ml APTT reagent
0.1 ml warmed kaolin suspension (after resuspension) and start stop watch.

The test tube is tilted three times immediately, and subsequently at approximately 1 min intervals in order to resuspend the kaolin.

At exactly 10 min 0.1 ml warmed calcium chloride (0.025 mol/L) is added. The tube is tilted gently three times and left undisturbed in a water bath for exactly 20 s from the addition of the calcium chloride. It is then tilted gently until a solid clot forms. The clotting time (seconds) is recorded and the test is performed in duplicate.

The normal range for the Manchester APTT is based on results from a large normal population of both sexes, spanning the adult age range. These extend from 36.0 to 48.0 s, based on two standard errors from the mean with correction for non-Gaussian distribution.

SOURCES OF ERROR

Although it is a relatively simple test to perform, the APTT is subject to a number of possible sources of error. The first can arise from faulty blood collection. Contamination by tissue juices, causing acceleration of the test, can result from traumatic and/or difficult venipuncture. In addition delay in mixing with the anticoagulant may cause partial clotting, which is not always obvious visually. In the ECAT studies this possibility has been minimized by the use of siliconized evacuated tubes. The use of test tubes for the performance of the test, which are not chemically clean, can also have a deleterious effect. With the manual technique, employed with the Manchester Reagent, it is important to control contact activation in order to facilitate the reading of the endpoint. During the incubation time the kaolin should be kept suspended in the reaction mixture by gentle mixing at regular intervals.

References

1. Stevenson KJ, Easton AC, Curry A, Thomson JM, Poller L. The reliability of activated partial thromboplastin time methods and the relationship to lipid composition and ultrastructure. Thromb Haemostas 1986; 55(2): 250–8.
2. Kelsey PR, Stevenson KJ, Poller L. The diagnosis of lupus anticoagulants by the activated partial thromboplastin time – The central role of phosphatidyl serine. Thromb Haemostas. 1984; 52: 172–5.
3. Barrowcliffe TW, Gray E. Studies of phospholipid reagents used in coagulation II: factors influencing their sensitivity to heparin. Thromb Haemostas 1981; 46(2): 634–7.
4. Thomson JM, Poller L. The activated partial thromboplastin time. In: Thomson JM., ed. Blood coagulation and haemostasis: a practical guide. Edinburgh: Churchill Livingstone, 1985; 301–39.
5. Triplett DA, Smith C. Sensitivity of the activated partial thromboplastin time: results of the CAP survey and a series of mild and moderate factor deficiencies. In: Triplett DA, ed. Standardisation of coagulation assays: an overview. Skokie, IL: College of American Pathologists, 1982; 137–63.
6. Koepke JA. The use of proficiency testing results in the coagulation laboratory. In: Triplett DA., ed., Laboratory evaluation of coagulation. Chicago, IL: American Society of Clinical Pathologists, 1982; 368–87.
7. Proctor RR, Rapaport SL. The partial thromboplastin time with kaolin. A simple screening test for first stage plasma clotting deficiencies. Am J Clin Pathol 1961; 36: 212–19.
8. Thomson JM. The control of heparin therapy by the activated partial thromboplastin time: sensitivity of various thromboplastins to heparin. In: Triplett DA, ed., Standardisation of coagulation assays: an overview. Skokie, IL: College of American Pathologists Press, 1982; 195–206.
9. Triplett DA. Heparin: Clinical use and monitoring. In: Triplett DA, ed., Laboratory evaluation of coagulation. Chicago, IL: American Society of Clinical Pathologists, 1982; 271–313.
10. Poller L, Thomson JM. The partial thromboplastin (cephalin) time test. J Clin Pathol 1972; 25: 1038–44.
11. Koepke J. The partial thromboplastin time in the CAP survey programme. Am J Clin Pathol 1974; 63: 990–4.
12. Shapiro GA, Huntzinger SW, Wilson JE. Variations among commercial activated partial thromboplastin time reagents in response to heparin. Am J Clin Pathol 1977; 67: 477–80.
13. CISMEL (Italian) Study Group. Activated partial thromboplastin time – a multi-centre evaluation of commercial reagents in the diagnosis of haemophilia. Scand J Haematol 1980; 25: 308.
14. Brandt JT, Triplett DA. Laboratory monitoring of heparin. Effect of reagents and instruments on the activated partial thromboplastin time. Am J Clin Pathol 1981; 76: 530–7.

15. Mannucci PM. A multicentre evaluation of partial thromboplastin time reagents in the detection of mild haemophiliacs. In: Triplett DM, ed., Standardisation of coagulation assays: an overview. Skokie, IL: College of American Pathologists, 1982; 165–77.
16. Hathaway WE, Bonnar J. Physiology of coagulation in the fetus and newborn infant. In: Perinatal coagulation. New York: Grune & Stratton, 1978; 69.

5
The prothrombin time test

L. POLLER

The prothrombin time (PT) is the screening test for the extrinsic (tissue) clotting system. The PT was originally introduced by Quick[1] as a measure of a coagulation defect in the newborn and jaundiced patients, and subsequently adapted for its present principal uses in the screening of extrinsic clotting and in monitoring of oral anticoagulant dosage. In the ECAT study we are concerned principally with its application in assessing extrinsic clotting function with emphasis on the screening of possible activation of the system in pre-thrombotic states. The PT reflects changes in three of the vitamin K-dependent clotting factors (factors II, VII and X), and the non-vitamin K-dependent factor V. The recalcification time of citrated plasma is accelerated in the PT by a tissue factor (TF) extract. The test depends on activation by TF of factor X in the presence of factor VII and the bypassing of the intrinsic pathway. The speed of this reaction and the responsiveness of the PT to deficiencies of clotting factors depends upon the properties and concentration of the TF.

SOURCES OF TISSUE EXTRACTS

Many modifications of the test have been introduced since Quick's original rabbit brain extract. Other tissues in addition to rabbit brain have been used as a source of TF in routine work, e.g. human brain, ox brain, monkey brain, rabbit lung and human placenta. TF is a combination of an apoprotein and phospholipid and is a complete thromboplastin as opposed to the partial thromboplastin of the APTT which lacks the apoprotein. It has been purified and its chemical structure has been defined[2,3]. Human recombinant TF is now being produced which when relipidated can be employed as the TF in the PT test[4,5]. This is still in the early stages, however, and until such material can be produced in large volumes, and shown to be satisfactory for routine

41

work, reliance will have to continue to be made on biological extracts. With present fears of virus transmission from human tissue the most widely used preparations are those derived from rabbit brain. These vary in their procoagulant properties and their ability to detect alterations in individual clotting factors or systems. The reagent adopted for the ECAT study is a responsive (low ISI) rabbit brain extract.

THE NORMAL RANGE AND THE EFFECT OF COAGULOMETERS

The normal range of the PT test varies with the different laboratory techniques. It is affected by the species of origin, tissue from which it is derived, the potency of the reagent as well as the local system of endpoint detection (i.e. whether manual or automated). The normal values for the PT test given with automated test systems are appreciably shorter than with the manual technique. The effects of coagulometers vary greatly not only between different brands of instrument but also to some extent between different coagulometers of the same model[6].

THE PT IN DIFFERENT CLINICAL STATES

The test is prolonged by oral anticoagulation, impairment of liver function, obstructive biliary disease and congenital deficiencies of factors II, V, VII and X. It is also prolonged by heparin administration although much less than is the APTT. The PT is considerably prolonged in the neonatal period and to a lesser extent throughout childhood. On the other hand, the PT may be accelerated in certain pre-thrombotic states, e.g. after administration of high-dose oestrogen oral contraceptives, after surgical operations and post-partum. In adult life there is a tendency to shortening of the test with increasing age.

LABORATORY VARIATION IN PT TESTING

The responsiveness of the PT test to a specific coagulation deficiency is dependent on the source and type of tissue thromboplastin. When the prothrombin time is used as a measure of the depression of vitamin K-dependent clotting factors, e.g. following oral anticoagulant administration or in liver function testing, the PT results with the different thromboplastins vary greatly. The overall sensitivity to the depression of factors II, VII and X during oral anticoagulant treatment is quantified numerically as the International Sensitivity Index (ISI) using the WHO international system of PT standardization[7-9]. This depends on a calibration of the individual thromboplastin extract against the WHO International Reference Preparation (IRP) for thromboplastin or a secondary IRP reagent calibrated in terms of the primary IRP. The responsiveness of the former is by definition 1.0. The slope of the orthogonal regression line when the log PT with the local thromboplastin of 20 normal and 60 coumarin-treated patients samples are plotted against those with an IRP indicates the responsiveness of the thromboplastin. This slope is defined as the ISI. Sensitive thromboplastins have an ISI value close to 1.0, whereas less responsive thromboplastins have higher values. Traditional North American reagents have ISI values between 2.0 and 2.8.

The use of a low ISI thromboplastin with good sensitivity to factor VII provides a reliable assessment of liver function. The progress of patients with liver disease and liver impairment secondary to other diseases and drug overdosages (e.g paracetamol, aspirin, etc.) may be monitored by the PT.

ECAT STUDY

A single recommended reagent and technique has been selected by the Executive Committee to be employed at all centres with a manual tilt tube technique. The manual method is recommended because coagulometers accelerate the test to varying degrees and may also affect the ISI.

The Manchester Reagent thromboplastin was selected for the ECAT study for several reasons. It has a low ISI (1.1 approximately) and shows good responsiveness to the individual extrinsic clotting factors and little interbatch variation. It has been shown to detect the acceleration of extrinsic clotting which occurs in the days following major surgery[10]. It shows good responsiveness to depession of factor VII in liver disease[11]. The precision of testing with Manchester Reagent in national external quality assessment has been shown to be greater than with some other reagents[12].

SOURCES OF ERROR

The test is relatively simple but subject to a number of pre-test and test variables which affect the result (see Chapter 2). Faulty blood collection and haemolysis affect the test. The use of siliconized or plastic test tubes instead of the recommended borosilicate glass tubes for the test, length and bore of glass tubes, angle and speed of the tilting are amongst the variables which affect the PT when performed manually.

TECHNIQUE

A standardized manual technique is provided therefore for the ECAT study as follows:

Prothrombin time test

Reagents

1   Calcium chloride 0.025 mol/l. Prepare from an M/1 solution. Store at 2–8° C.
2   Thromboplastin, Manchester Reagent. Store at 2–8 °C. *Do not freeze.*

Method

N.B.: A manual (tilt-tube) technique must be used.

Testing should be performed as soon as possible after collection, preferably within 1 h from venipuncture. Maintain plasma in a stoppered polystyrene container at room temperature.

Warm sufficient test tubes for performance of the test in a 37°C water bath (tolerance limits 37.0 ± 0.2 °C). Clean, new glass tubes should be used.

1 Resuspend the thromoplastin extract by gentle inversion and transfer 0.1 vol into glass test tubes in the water bath. Allow to warm for 1–2 min. Thromboplastin should not be allowed to pre-warm in the test tubes for > 1 h.

2 Add 0.1 ml plasma using automatic pipette. New pipetting tips must be used for each plasma.

3 After approximately 1 min add 0.1 ml pre-warmed calcium chloride (0.025 mol/l) and start stopwatch.

   Tilt gently, keeping tubes under water as much as possible to maintain optimal temperature. The speed and angle of tilting the test tube must be standardized (three tilts through 90° every 5 s) to control glass activation and minimize cooling. Record endpoint in clotting time (seconds).

Tests should be performed in duplicate. If the discrepancy between duplicate tests is more than 5% of the mean clotting time the test should be repeated, i.e. if the mean clotting time is 30 s, duplicates should range between 28.5 and 31.5 s.

References

1. Quick J. The prothrombin time in haemophilia and in obstructive jaundice. J Biol Chem 1935; 109: 73–4.
2. Broze GJ, Leykam JE, Schwartz BD, Miletich JP. Purification of human brain tissue. J Biol Chem 1985; 260: 10917–20.
3. Guha A, Bach R, Konigsberg W, Nemerson Y. Affinity purification of human tissue factor: interaction of factor VII and tissue factor in detergent micelles. Proc Natl Acad Sci USA 1986; 299–302.
4. Morrissey JH, Fair DS, Edgington TS. Structure and properties of the human tissue factor apoprotein. Thromb Haemostas 1987; 58: 257.
5. Fujikawa K, Suzuki K. Cellular coagulant and anticoagulant proteins. In: Poller A, ed. Recent advances in blood coagulation, vol. 5. London: Churchill Livingstone, 1991; 35–51.
6. Thomson JM, Taberner DA, Poller L. Automation and the prothrombin time: a United Kingdom field study of two widely used coagulometers. J Clin Pathol 1990; 43: 679–84.
7. Kirkwood TBL. Calibration of reference thromboplastins. Thromb Haemostas 1983; 49: 238–44.
8. Hermans J, Van den Besselaar AMHP, Loeliger EA, Van der Velde EA. A collaborative calibration study of reference materials for thromboplastins. Thromb Haemostas 1983; 50: 712–7.
9. Thomson JM, Tomenson JA, Poller L. The calibration of the Second Primary International Reference Preparation for Thromboplastin (thromboplastin, human, plain, coded BCT/253). Thromb Haemostas 1984; 52: 336–42.

10. Poller L, McKernan A, Thomson JM, Elstein M, Hirsh PJ, Jones PB. Fixed minidose warfarin: a new approach to prophylaxis against venous thrombosis after major surgery. Br Med J 1987; 295: 1309–12.
11. Kitchen S, Malia RG, Greaves M, Preston FE: Comparison of human and rabbit brain thromboplastin in evaluation of haemostatic defect of liver disease. Lancet 1986; 2: 1463.
12. Taberner DA, Poller L, Thomson JM, Darby KV. Effect of International Sensitivity Index (ISI) of thromboplastins on precision of International Normalised Ratio (INR). J Clin Pathol 1989; 42: 92–100.

6
Fibrinogen

G. A. MARBET and F. DUCKERT

INTRODUCTION

Blood coagulation ultimately depends on the thrombin-induced conversion of fibrinogen to fibrin[1-3]. Fibrinogen is a dimeric symmetric macromolecule. Each half consists of three different polypeptide chains, Aα, Bβ and γ, linked together by disulphide bridges. The two sets of chains are connected at the aminoterminal end region by three disulphide bridges, two between the γ-chains and one between the α-chains. This native fibrinogen of 340 kD molecular weight (high molecular weight fibrinogen HMW fbg) is primarily the substrate of thrombin action resulting in the release of both fibrinopeptide A and fibrinopeptide B from the aminoterminal end. Less specific cleavages of fibrinogen may occur *in vivo*[3]. Extensive fibrinogenolysis mainly occurs during treatment with streptokinase or urokinase. Even the plasma of normal donors shows some evidence of fibrinogen cleavage[4,5]. Low molecular weight fibrinogens, LMWfbg of about 305 kD and LMW'fbg of about 270 kD, result from the removal of a 35 kD carboxyterminal polypeptide from one Aα-chain and from both Aα-chains respectively[6,7]. The identity of proteolytic enzymes responsible for the *in vivo* generation of LMW fbg under physiological conditions is at present uncertain.

According to Holm and Godal[6] the physiological distribution of heterogeneous fibrinogens is 69.7%, 26.5% and 3.8% for HMW, LMW and LMW'fbg respectively[6]. This distribution has been confirmed by Furlan *et al.*[8]. The clotting times of the degraded fibrinogens are prolonged[7,9].

Fibrinogen is necessary for clot formation and appropriate platelet function *in vivo*. Its normal plasma level ranges between 1.7 and 4.0 g/L, corresponding to 5–12 μmol/L. The Michaelis–Menten constant K_m for the cleavage of the Aα-chain[10-13] by thrombin is about 7 μmol/L. Therefore, the velocity of clot formation is significantly affected by different fibrinogen concentrations even within the 'physiological' range. This is one biochemical component of the

47

increased thrombotic risk associated with higher plasma fibrinogen concentration.

Fibrinogen is involved as an important pathophysiological variable in various clinicopathological conditions[1-3], e.g. disseminated intravascular coagulation (DIC), liver disease, thrombolytic therapy, infection, malignancy and obstetric emergencies. Therefore, its measurement is often required by the clinician as an emergency test.

Clinical disorders that regularly raise fibrinogen and other acute-phase proteins usually exhibit a higher frequency of thromboembolic complications. Oral contraceptive drugs also induce elevated fibrinogen levels[21-23] even if their oestrogen content is low[23].

In addition epidemiological studies have been accumulating convincing evidence for several decades[14-20] that fibrinogen is an independent risk factor of cardiovascular morbidity. The association of smoking with coronary artery disease may to some extent be mediated by increased fibrinogen levels[14,15,18].

METHOD OF FIBRINOGEN ASSAY

Numerous methods have been published for the determination of fibrinogen in plasma[24]. They are based on different principles: heat or salt precipitation[25], total clottable protein[26-28], thrombin clotting rate assays[29,30], turbidimetry and light scattering of clotting plasma[31-36] and immunological techniques[36]. Assays measuring total clottable fibrinogen have been used for decades to calibrate the more practical clotting rate assays or their turbidimetric equivalents. Immunological assays of functional fibrinogen require multiple steps: clot formation, careful washing to remove pre-existing fibrin(ogen) degradation products, then clot digestion by plasmin and electroimmunoassay with anti-fibrinogen antibodies[37].

Principle and assay characteristics (clotting rate assay)

The chronometric assay by Clauss[29] is based on the clotting time of a mixture of diluted plasma and a standardized thrombin solution. The recorded clotting times depend on the plasma concentration of functional fibrinogen. The plasma dilution reduces the influence of inhibitors, i.e. heparin, but not the retarding effects of fibrin(ogen) degradation products. The fibrinogen values in g/L are obtained by comparing the clotting times of unknown plasma samples with serial dilutions of a reference plasma with known fibrinogen concentration according to bioassay principles.

Materials (clotting rate assay)

Isotonic barbital-acetate buffer pH 7.35 (BAB)

1. *Stock solution*: 9.714 g sodium acetate. $3 H_2O$ and 14.714 g sodium 5,5-diethylbarbiturate in 500 ml distilled water.

2. *Working solution (barbital-acetate buffer BAB)*: 250 ml stock solution, 200 ml NaCl 4.25%, 217 ml HCl 0.1 mol/L and 683 ml distilled water. The pH may be corrected with very slight amounts of HCl.

Thrombin stock solution

This solution and all thrombin dilutions are prepared with plastic material or well-siliconized glassware. Thrombin Roche or Topostasin Roche is dissolved in BAB to a final concentration of 800 U/ml. This solution remains at 2 °C for 2 h until complete dissolution. Then the same volume of sterile, water-free glycerol is added and carefully mixed. This solution contains 400 U/ml thrombin and is stable for months at −20 °C. When using the Kabi or other thrombin preparations their stock solution diluted 1:80 should give an average clotting time of 15 s (13−17 s) with citrated plasma of normal individuals in the following assay at 37 °C.

    0.2 ml normal plasma
            incubate 30 s at 37 °C, add
    0.1 ml thrombin solution
            record clotting

Thrombin working solution

Before use the thrombin solution is diluted 1:12 with BAB (1 part thrombin stock solution + 11 parts BAB). It is necessary to make sure that the stock solution is homogeneous and gently tilt the bottle before pipetting the desired amount. The solution is viscous and pipetting must be performed carefully in order to guarantee day-to-day reproducibility. After filling the pipette the tip is carefully cleaned with soft wiping tissue to eliminate excess solution adhering to the external surface of the tip. This diluted working solution is stable at 2−4 °C for 2 h.

Procedure

Citrated plasma is used for the assay. The plasma to be tested is diluted 1:10 with BAB immediately before the assay. Note that 1:10 dilution corresponds to 1 part plasma in 10 parts of the *mixture*; in other words to 1 part of plasma 9 parts of BAB are added = 10 parts of mixture.

    0.1 ml 1:10 diluted citrated plasma
            after 30 s incubation at 37 °C add
    0.1 ml thrombin solution 33 U/ml

Record the clotting time, using Kolle hook and a stopwatch or a coagulometer.

Evaluation of results

The calibration curve of the Clauss assay is obtained from the clotting times of serial dilutions (1:10, 1:20, 1:30, 1:50) of a standard plasma with known clottable fibrinogen concentration. Double logarithmic paper is used to plot times on the ordinate against the concentrations (g/L) on the abscissa. The clotting times of the diluted test plasma samples are then converted into fibrinogen concentrations. The shape of the calibration curve depends on the method used to detect the clotting endpoints. In our hands it was hyperbolic with the hook method and linear with the KC-10 coagulometer in the log–log plot (Figure 6.1).

The fibrinogen concentration assigned to some commercial reference plasmas may be doubtful (see p. 52). They can be checked by some reliable assay of total clottable fibrinogen[8,26,28]. For our calibration curve we use five to 10 different plasmas with clottable fibrinogen determined by the Blombäck method[28] briefly described on pp. 52–3.

Precision and reliability of the clotting rate assay

Each test is done in duplicate and must be repeated if the clotting times differ by more than 1.0 s. Appropriate measurements can be obtained only within the range of 0.8–8.0 g/L of the calibration curve. Greater plasma dilutions

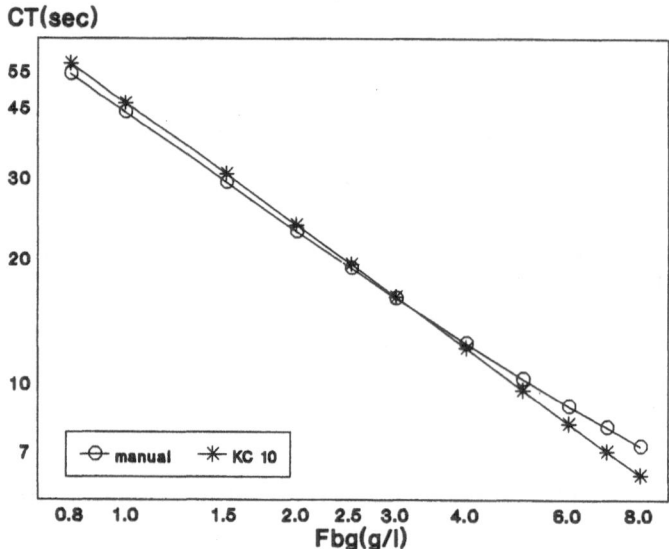

Figure 6.1 Reference curves of the clotting rate assay by Clauss. ○, Curve with *manual* endpoint (hook method), approximated by equation $CT = A/[\text{fbg}] + B$, where CT = Clauss clotting time (s), [fbg] = fibrinogen concentration (g/L); A and B are curve parameters. $A = 41.29 \pm 2.32$ and $B = 2.16 \pm 0.28$ (mean ± SD) from eight curves with different lots of bovine thrombin (Roche) and reference plasmas (1982–90). *, Curve with KC 10 according to the equation $^{10}\log CT = a \times {}^{10}\log [\text{fbg}] + b$. The parameters of six calibration curves obtained from different lots were (mean ± SD): $a = -0.9573 \pm 0.0167$ and $b = 1.6610 \pm 0.0152$.

(1:20, 1:30 or 1:40) may be required for high fibrinogen values. Vice-versa, values below 0.8 g/L should be repeated with a 1:5 plasma dilution. For the calculation of the results any deviation from the regular 1:10 plasma dilution must be taken into account by the appropriate multiplication factor. In the Basle clinical coagulation laboratory the coefficients of variation from day to day are 3–5% in the fibrinogen range of 2–4 g/L, in accordance with published results of the ECAT Angina Pectoris Study[38].

Excessive heparin levels (>0.8 U/ml) may give falsely low fibrinogen values. Clauss fibrinogen is usually lower than total clottable or immunologically measured fibrinogen in conditions with increased fibrin(ogen) degradation products such as disseminated intravascular coagulation and therapeutic fibrinolysis. This also occurs in dysfibrinogenaemia with slowly clotting abnormal fibrinogen[3,39].

Reference values

The normal range of plasma fibrinogen with the Clauss method is 1.7–4.0 g/L. The distribution of these values is skewed to the right.

Calibration and commercial fibrinogen standards

The calibration of plasma fibrinogen determinations is hampered by the absence of an international fibrinogen standard. In a careful study of 10 commercially available fibrinogen standards Furlan et al.[8] found deviations up to 80% of the declared from the measured clottable fibrinogen content. With the availability of an international reference preparation the calibration of commercial fibrinogen standards will certainly improve.

In our laboratory the assay of total clottable fibrinogen by Blombäck and Blombäck[28] is applied to measure the content of functional fibrinogen in plasma samples serving as standards for the calibration curve of the clotting rate assay by Clauss[29].

An alternative method for total clottable fibrinogen has been described by Ratnoff and Menzie[26] and modified by Swain and Feders[27].

Principle and assay characteristics of the Blombäck and Blombäck method[28]

The fibrinogen is separated from other plasma proteins by clotting diluted plasma, eliminating the soluble proteins by gently expressing the serum with subsequent washing of the clot. The long incubation time after addition of thrombin allows a quantitative fibrin formation. Epsilon aminocaproic acid is added to avoid any fibrinolytic dissolution of the clot. Because of the long incubation time the clot includes, besides fibrin, the larger degradation products of fibrin(ogen) present in the plasma. Some traces of other proteins may remain trapped in the clot. This explains why in abnormal plasmas (especially when the fibrinolytic system is active) the values found with the

Blombäck and Blombäck assay are higher (additional material included in the clot) than with the Clauss assay (inhibiting effect of FDP).

The fibrinogen is converted to fibrin with thrombin without Ca^{2+} ions. Therefore, the clot is not stabilized and remains soluble in concentrated urea. The fibrinogen concentration can be measured either by determination of the tyrosine in the well-washed clot or more easily by measuring the light absorbance at 282 nm.

Materials and assay procedure are given in Tables 6.1 and 6.2 respectively.

Correlation with various assay modifications

The clotting rate assay[29] is influenced by large amounts of intermediate and late FDPs. In DIC and under thrombolytic therapy it may underestimate the 'true' level of clottable fibrinogen[3,35,36,40-43]; but its value is a clinically appropriate indicator of the clotting defect.

With increasing automation of the clinical coagulation laboratory various adaptations of functional assays have been proposed. Fibrin polymerization is induced by thrombin[33-36,43] or by batroxobin[31,32] and recorded by various optical methods. With normal plasma the agreement between manually performed clotting rate assays[29,30] or total clottable fibrinogen[26,27,28] and the automated tests is acceptable.

Discordant results were reported for plasma samples of patients with DIC, thrombolytic therapy, heparin treatment or hyperlipaemia[34-36].

Such systematic differences may depend on the way the analyser recognizes fibrin polymerization. The photometric assessment of increasing turbidity (change of absorbance per minute at 334 nm) after addition of batroxobin has successfully been used in a centrifugal analyser[32]. The test system is somewhat less affected by elevated fibrin(ogen) degradation products than the manual clotting rate assay, but influenced by high plasma turbidity[31,32]. Photo-optical clot detection and registration of the clotting time by another analyser apparently reached excellent agreement with the Clauss assay on

Table 6.1 Materials used for the Blombäck and Blombäck Method[28]

Phosphate buffer
55.5 mol of 0.2 mol/L KH_2PO_4 (27.218 g/L), 7.2 ml of 0.2 mol/L $Na_2HPO_4 \cdot 2H_2O$ (35.598 g/L) and H_2O added up to a volume of 100 ml, pH = 5.9, ionic strength 0.15, molarity 0.125

Epsilon aminocaproic acid (EACA)
10% EACA in distilled water

Thrombin solution (Thrombin Roche)
100 NIH U/ml in phosphate buffer pH 5.9. The solution is kept in plastic or well-siliconized glassware

Alkaline urea solution (40%)
Solution of 6.7 mol/L urea and 0.2 mol/L NaOH, mix 400 g urea and 8 g NaOH in 1000 ml H_2O

Glass tube 14 mm diameter and 9.5 cm in length

Nylon tissue 180×180 mesh/cm^2

Plasmas
Five to 10 different plasma samples, some with high fibrinogen concentrations

---

Table 6.2 Performance of the Blombäck and Blombäck Assay[28]

Assay mixture
0.3 ml plasma
0.75 ml phosphate buffer
0.195 ml EACA
0.075 ml Thrombin
are rapidly and thoroughly mixed and left at room temperature for 2 h

1. A piece of the nylon tissue is placed on top of a layer of a very absorbent soft wiping tissue or cellulose tissue
2. The incubation mixture with the clot is carefully poured on the nylon, the solution is absorbed by the tissue underneath
3. After retraction the clot is washed three times with 0.9% NaCl. Change absorbing tissue each time. *The clot should never become dry. Do not lose small pieces of the clot.* Washing is the most difficult step of the assay
4. After washing, transfer clot to a tube containing 2.5 ml alkaline urea solution and incubate 5–10 min at room temperature. Then the clots are gently shaken until complete dissolution after about 2 h
5. The extinction E is measured at 282 nm in a quartz cuvette, 1 cm lightpath using the alkaline urea solution as a blank

The fibrinogen concentration (fbg) is calculated according to the following formula for 0.3 ml plasma:

$$E \times U/(E_{1\,cm}^{0.1\%} \times V) = E/0.198 = \text{fbg (g/L)}$$

where $E_{1\,cm}^{0.1\%}$ at 282 nm $= 1.65$, $U =$ urea volume (2.5 ml), $V =$ plasma volume (0.3 ml). The absorbance values are stable for 24 h

---

the KC 10 coagulometer[33]. Discrepancies have been observed with analysers monitoring thrombin-induced fibrin polymerization by light scattering[34–36,43]. Spuriously high fibrinogen values under thrombolytic therapy or in DIC may be misleading for the clinician.

Clotting rate assays of fibrinogen performed on automatic analysers should therefore be systematically compared with manual techniques on both normal and pathological samples.

References

1. Doolittle RF. Fibrinogen and fibrin. In: Bloom AL, Thomas DP, eds. Haemostasis and thrombosis. Edinburgh: Churchill Livingstone, 1987; 192–215.
2. Hantgan RR, Francis DW, Scheraga HA, Marder VJ. Fibrinogen structure and physiology. In: Colman RW, Hirsh J, Marder VJ, Salzman EW, eds. Hemostasis and thrombosis, 2nd ed. Philadelphia: Lippincott, 1987; 269–88.
3. Francis CW, Marder VJ. Physiologic regulation and pathologic disorders of fibrinolysis. In: Colman RW, Hirsh J, Marder VJ, Salzman EW, eds. Hemostasis and thrombosis, 2nd ed. Philadelphia: Lippincott, 1987; 358–79.
4. Mosesson MW, Finlayson JS, Umfleet RA, Galanakis D. Human fibrinogen heterogeneities. I. Structural and related studies of plasma fibrinogens which are high solubility catabolic intermediates. J Biol Chem 1972; 247: 5210–19.
5. Lipinska I, Lipinski B, Gurewich V. Fibrinogen heterogeneity in human plasma. Electrophoretic demonstration and chracterization of two major fibrinogen components. J Lab Clin Med 1974; 84: 509–16.
6. Holm B, Godal HC. Quantitation of three normally occurring plasma fibrinogens in health

and during so-called 'acute phase' by SDS electrophoresis of fibrin obtained from EDTA-plasma. Thromb Res 1984; 35: 279–90.

7. Holm B, Nilsen DWT, Kierulf P, Godal HC. Purification and characterization of 3 fibrinogens with different molecular weights obtained from normal human plasma. Thromb Res 1985; 37: 165–76.

8. Furlan M, Felix R, Escher N, Lämmle B. How high is the true fibrinogen content of fibrinogen standards? Thromb Res 1989; 56: 583–92.

9. Holm B, Brosstad F, Kierulf P, Godal HC. Polymerization properties of two normally circulating fibrinogens, HMW and LMW. Evidence that the COOH-terminal end of the a-chain is of importance for fibrin polymerization. Thromb Res 1985; 39: 595–606.

10. Bando M, Matsushima A, Hirano J, Imadu Y. Thrombin-catalyzed conversion of fibrinogen to fibrin. J Biochem 1972; 71: 897–9.

11. Martinelli RA, Scheraga HA. Steady-state kinetic study of the bovine thrombin-fibrinogen interaction. Biochemistry 1980; 19: 2343–50.

12. Higgins DL, Lewis SD, Shafer JA. Steady state kinetic parameters for the thrombin catalyzed conversion of human fibrinogen to fibrin. J Biol Chem 1983; 258: 9276–82.

13. Lewis SD, Shafer JA. A thrombin assay based upon the release of fibrinopeptide A from fibrinogen: definition of a new thrombin unit. Thromb Res 1984; 35: 111–20.

14. Wilhelmsen L, Svardsudd K, Korsan-Bengtsen K, Larsson B, Welin L. Tibblin G. Fibrinogen as a risk factor for stroke and myocardial infarction. N Engl J Med 1984; 311: 501–5.

15. Korsan-Bengtsen K, Wilhelmsen L, Tibblin G. Blood coagulation and fibrinolysis in a random sample of 788 men 54 years old: Relations of the variables to 'risk factors' for myocardial infarction. Thromb Diathes Haemorrh 1972; 28: 99–108.

16. Meade TW, North WRS, Chakrabarti R, Stirling Y, Haines AP, Thompson SG. Haemostatic function and cardiovascular death: early results of a prospective study. Lancet 1980; 1: 1050–4.

17. Meade TW, Mellows S, Brozovic M, Miller SG, Chakrabarti RR, North WRS, Haines AP, Stirling Y, Imeson ID, Thomson SG. Haemostatic function and ischaemic heart disease: Principal results of the Northwich Park Heart Study. Lancet 1986; 2: 533–7.

18. Meade TW. The epidemiology of haemostatic and other variables in coronary artery disease. In: Verstraete M, Vermylen J, Lijnen HR, Arnout J, eds. Thrombosis and haemostasis. Leuven University Press, 1987; 37–60.

19. Stone MC, Thorpe JM. Plasma fibrinogen – a major coronary risk factor. J R Coll Gen Pract 1985; 36: 565–9.

20. Kannel WB, Wolf PA, Castelli WP, D'Agostino RB. Fibrinogen and risk of cardiovascular disease. The Framingham Study. J Am Med Assoc 1987; 258: 1183–6.

21. Meade TW, Brozovic M, Chakrabarti R, Howarth DJ, North WRS, Stirling Y. An epidemiological study of the haemostatic and other effects of oral contraceptives. Br J Haematol 1976; 34: 353–64.

22. Poller L. Oral contraceptives, blood clotting and thrombosis. Br Med Bull 1978; 34: 151–6.

23. Toulon P, Bardin JM, Blumenfeld N. Increased heparin cofactor II levels in women taking oral contraceptives. Thromb Haemostas 1990; 64: 365–8.

24. Exner T, Burridge J, Power P, Rickard KA. An evaluation of currently available methods for plasma fibrinogen. Am J Clin Pathol 1979; 71: 521–7.

25. Schulz FH. Eine einfache Bewertungsmethode von Leberparenchymschäden (volumetrische Fibrinbestimmung). Acta Hepatol 1955; 3: 306–10.

26. Ratnoff OD, Menzie C. A new method for the determination of fibrinogen in small samples of plasma. J Lab Clin Med 1951; 37: 316–20.

27. Swain W, Feders MB. Fibrinogen assay. Clin Chem 1967; 13: 1026–8.

28. Blombäck B, Blombäck M. Preparation of human fibrinogen fraction 1–2. Arkiv Kemi 1956; 10: 415–43.

29. Clauss A. Gerinnungsphysiologische Schnellmethode zur Bestimmung des Fibrinogens. Acta Haematol 1957; 17: 237–46.

30. Vermylen C, de Vreker RA, Verstraete M. A rapid enzymatic method for assay of fibrinogen fibrin polymerization time (FPT Test). Clin Chim Acta 1963; 8: 418–24.

31. Becker U, Bartl K, Wahlefeld AW. A functional photometric assay for plasma fibrinogen. Thromb Res 1984; 35: 475–84.

32. De Metz M, van Wersch JWJ. Use of a centrifugal analyzer for a chromogenic prothrombin time, a chromogenic activated partial thromboplastin time and a kinetic fibrinogen assay

in a routine hospital laboratory. Haemostasis 1987; 17: 254–9.

33. Cambas JP, Biermé R, Martinon JC, Dousset B. Evaluation des performances d'un automate en coagulation: l'Electra 700 Nouv Rev Fr Hematol 1985; 25: 313–20.

34. Bick RZ, Wheeler A, Camposano N. A comparative study of the DuPont antithrombin III and fibrinogen assay systems. Am J Clin Pathol 1985; 83: 541–6.

35. Hoffman M, Greenberg CS. The effects of fibrin polymerization inhibitors on quantitative measurements of plasma fibrinogen. Am J Clin Pathol 1987; 88: 490–3.

36. Hoffmann JJML, Verhappen MAL. Automated nephelometry of fibrinogen: Analytical performance and observations during thrombolytic therapy. Clin Chem 1988; 34: 2135–40.

37. Laurell CB. Quantitative estimation of proteins by electrophoresis in agarose gel containing antibodies. Anal Biochem 1966; 15: 45–52.

38. Thompson SG, Duckert F, Haverkate F, Thomson JM. The measurement of haemostatic factors in 15 European laboratories: Quality assessment for the multicentre ECAT Angina pectoris study. Thromb Haemostas 1989; 61: 301–6.

39. McDonagh J, Carrell N. Disorders of fibrinogen structure and function. In: Colman RW, Hirsh J, Marder VJ, Salzman EW, eds. Hemostasis and thrombosis, 2nd ed. Philadelphia: Lippincott, 1987; 301–17.

40. Marder VJ, Shulman NR. High molecular weight derivatives of human fibrinogen produced by plasmin. II. Mechanism of their anticoagulant activity. J Biol Chem 1969; 244: 2120–4.

41. Saleem A, Fretz K. An improved method for plasma fibrinogen based on thrombin time measurement. Clin Chim Acta 1975; 62: 131–6.

42. Jespersen J, Sidelmann JA. A study of the conditions and accuracy of the thrombin time assay of plasma fibrinogen. Acta Haematol 1982; 67: 2–7.

43. Lurie AA, Gross LF, Rogers WJ. The measurement of fibrinogen by the DuPont aca and Dade methods in patients receiving streptokinase infusions. Am J Clin Pathol 1985; 84: 526–9.

7
Factor VII clotting activity

G. A. MARBET and F. DUCKERT

INTRODUCTION

Factor VII is a single-chain, vitamin K-dependent glycoprotein of molecular weight 47 000–50 000[1–5]. Its plasma concentration is about 250–700 ng/ml (5–15 nmol/L). The complex of the zymogen factor VII with tissue thromboplastin and Ca^{2+} has been proposed as an efficient activator of factor X[7,8]. Factor VII can be converted to the two-chain α-VIIa by hydrolysis of an Arg–Ile bond by factors Xa, IXa, XIIa or thrombin[1,2,6,10]. The coagulant activity of α-VIIa is 100-fold increased compared to single-chain factor VII[8]. Further cleavage of α-VIIa at the heavy chain destroys coagulant activity[9]. The complex of factor VII/VIIa with tissue factor also activates factor IX to IXa[11,12]. Some authors[13,14] virtually deny any physiologically relevant enzymatic activity to the complex of tissue factor with non-activated factor VII. Their concept of extrinsic activation requires the presence of factor VIIa in trace amounts. Factor Xa will then be generated by the factor VIIa/tissue factor complex (and also by reactions of the intrinsic coagulation pathway) and activate the thromboplastin bound zymogen factor VII to VIIa. This potent amplification loop is subjected to complex regulation mechanisms[15].

Factor VII as the only coagulation factor of the extrinsic pathway is relevant for normal haemostasis. Patients with severe congenital deficiency suffer from spontaneous bleeding of joints and mucosal membranes[16,17].

Factor VII has the shortest plasma half-life of all coagulation factors. Its coagulant activity decreases rapidly within a few hours after the start of administration of vitamin K antagonists. Epidemiological studies have demonstrated a positive association between increased factor VII:C levels and cardiovascular morbidity[18–21]. This may partly be due to an increased proportion of circulating α-VIIa resulting in an excess of factor VII coagulant activity over factor VII antigen[21–27]. α-Factor VIIa formation in citrated plasma can be enhanced in glass tubes by exposure to 0–4 °C over a period of several hours[22].

This 'cold activation phenomenon' can easily be induced in plasma of women on oral contraceptive drugs or during pregnancy[28–30,33].

METHOD OF ASSAY

The conventional methods to quantitate factor VII clotting activity in plasma (VII:C) are clotting rate assays. Diluted test plasma is added to a substrate plasma specifically deficient in factor VII activity and the clotting time of the mixture is measured after activation by tissue thromboplastin and calcium chloride. The clotting times of the test sample are compared to those of the dilution of a normal pool plasma. The potency estimation follows the rules of the parallel line assay[31,32].

Critical reagents

As congenital factor VII deficiency is rare only a few reliable factor VII-deficient substrate plasmas are commercially available. Therefore, factor VII immune-depleted plasma may also be used as a substrate[33–36]. It may even be superior to some congenitally deficient plasmas still containing factor VII antigen and variable levels of residual factor VII activity depending on the type of thromboplastin used[33,35]. The sensitivity of the test system (slope of the standard curve) is also a function of the source of the tissue thromboplastin used.

In this respect human thromboplastin may be preferred[33,35]. Plasma of congenitally factor VII-deficient dogs has also successfully been used as a substrate instead of human deficiency plasma[37–39]. For the analysis of plasma samples of the ECAT Angina Pectoris Study we had the opportunity to use factor VII-deficient plasma of beagle dogs from the UK Reference Laboratory in Manchester[39] and our home-made human brain tissue thromboplastin. In our laboratory this assay system has been sensitive to 'cold activation' of factor VII.

Materials

1. Factor VII-deficient plasma, possible sources: (a) Commercially available congenitally deficient plasma without any detectable factor VII activity (checked in a test system with human tissue thromboplastin as an activator). (b) Immune-depleted factor VII free normal human plasma. (c) Canine factor VII-deficient plasma[39] from the UK Reference Laboratory for Anticoagulant Reagents and Quality Control, batches No. 138, 152, 301 have been used in the ECAT Angina Pectoris Study.
2. Test plasma obtained from citrated blood, snap-frozen and stored at −70 °C.
3. Normal reference plasma obtained by pooling of equal amounts of plasma from 40–60 healthy volunteers. Aliquots (0.5 ml) of mixed plasma are snap-frozen and stored in liquid nitrogen.

4. Veronal acetate buffer (VAB) for plasma dilution (see Chapter 6).
5. Human brain thromboplastin, prepared from acetone brain dry powder and diluted in saline to obtain thromboplastin times of 11–13 s with a normal plasma pool of 43 male donors. The thromboplastin suspension in saline was stored at $-70\,°C$ before use.

   Commercially available thromboplastin of human origin: Thromborel S (Behringwerke Marburg). Thromboplastin preparations of animal origin together with immune-depleted human plasma in the test system are also sensitive to activated factor VII[33].
6. Calcium chloride, 25 mmol/L in distilled H_2O.
7. KC-10 coagulometer from Amelung, or any other device able to detect the clotting endpoint accurately and reproducibly.

Procedure

For each assay series a standard curve is made at the beginning and at the end. Activities are defined by dilutions of the reference plasma in VAB: 1:10 (100%), 1:20 (50%), 1:40 (25%), 1:80 (12.5%). Test plasma is diluted with VAB 1:20 or more in non-anticoagulated cases and 1:10 in patients on oral anticoagulants. Each test is performed in duplicate in the following order:

Factor VII-deficient plasma at 22 °C   100 μl
Diluted plasma sample at 22 °C   100 μl
Human brain thromboplastin at 37 °C   100 μl

Incubation time at 37 °C for 20 s

$CaCl_2$ sol. 25 mmol/L at 37 °C   100 μl
Clotting time on KC 10

Evaluation of results

The standard curve represented by a double logarithmic plot of clotting times versus percentage activities is a straight line. It is used for the conversion of the clotting times of the test plasma samples into factor VII activity. For the final result predilution has to be considered.

Reproducibility

The reproducibility of the standard curves from day to day is quite satisfactory with identical batches of canine factor VII-deficient plasma and human thromboplastin. Slope and Y-intercepts are shown in Table 7.1 for three different batches of canine substrate plasma used at different times with different batches of human brain thromboplastin. Between batches the curve parameters differ significantly. The slopes are steeper than corresponding values reported by Brandt et al.[33]. The within-assay variation at the level of 70% and 20% activity is satisfactory with a coefficiency variation (CV) of 4–5%.

Table 7.1 Standard curves of VII:C-assay – log (seconds) vs log (per cent)

Batch no.	n	Slope	Y-Intercept
138	9	−0.268 (0.007)	1.726 (0.011)
152	2	−0.243 (0.007)	1.699 (0.011)
301	28	−0.216 (0.004)	1.624 (0.007)

n = Number of standard curves; standard deviation in parentheses.

Despite the good reproducibility of the standard curves the between-day CV easily exceeds the level of 10% for VII:C < 50%. This is also known from other clotting assays with relatively flat slopes such as factor V, VIII and IX [41-43]. In our experience the between-assay variation was not smaller with a human factor VII-deficient plasma despite the steeper reference curves (average slope −0.412).

Factor VII:C level

In healthy men and in non-pregnant women without oral contraceptive drugs the factor VII:C level is 70–130%. This corresponds with reported ranges in healthy normals[5,33,34,45].

Factor VII standard

No international factor VII standard is yet available. Quality control has to be based on home-made 'normal' and 'abnormal' (usually from patients on oral anticoagulants) deep-frozen control plasmas or from commercially available lyophilized material. Non-activating plastic tubes should be used to store test, control and internal standard plasmas and any prolonged exposure to temperatures of 0–4 °C should be avoided by snap-freezing and rapid thawing.

Factor VII levels in plasma

These can also be measured with amidolytic (VII am) and immunological assays (VII:Ag). In the amidolytic assay[26,27,33,35,44] factor VII is entirely activated into α-VIIa and then factor Xa formation is measured with a chromogenic substrate. This test detects the total of functional factor VII coagulant activity and is insensitive to variable ratios of single-chain factor VII and two-chain (preactivated) α-VIIa.

The immunological assays, radioligand assays (RIA/IRMA) and enzyme-linked immunosorbent assays (ELISA)[25,35,45-47] detect coagulant-active and inactive forms of plasma factor VII. The use of amidolytic and/or immunological assays, together with the clotting assay, has been rewarding for the characterization of congenital and acquired factor VII deficiency[33,35,47]. The ratio between VII:C and VII am or VII:Ag may be quite sensitive to preactivation of factor VII *in vivo* and reflects the presence of an increased thrombotic risk[22-25,27,48].

If only one factor VII assay can be performed in an epidemiological study in order to evaluate its relevance as a risk factor for thromboembolism the clotting test will be preferred.

References

1. Broze GJ, Majerus PW. Purification and properties of human coagulation factor VII. J Biol Chem 1980; 255: 1242–7.
2. Bajaj SP, Rapaport SI, Brown SF. Isolation and chracterization of human factor VII. Activation of factor VII by factor Xa. J Biol Chem 1981; 256: 253–9.
3. Radcliffe RD, Nemerson Y. The activation and control of factor VII by activated factor X and thrombin. J Biol Chem 1975; 250: 338–95.
4. Broze GJ, Majerus PW. Human VII. Meth Enzymol 1982; 80: 228–34.
5. Fair DS. Quantitation of factor VII in the plasma of normal and warfarin-treated individuals by radioimmunoassay. Blood 1983; 62: 784–91.
6. Masys DR, Bajaj SP, Rapaport SI. Activation of human factor VII by activated factors IX and X. J Biol Chem 1981; 256: 253–9.
7. Radcliffe R, Nemerson Y. Activation and control of factor X and thrombin: Isolation and characterization of a high chain form of factor VII. J Biol Chem 1972; 250: 388–95.
8. Bach R, Oberdick J, Nemerson Y. Immunoaffinity purification of bovine factor VII. Blood 1984; 63: 393–8.
9. Radcliffe R, Nemerson Y. Mechanism of action of bovine factor VII: Products of cleavage by factor Xa. J Biol Chem 1976; 251: 4797–802.
10. Radcliffe RD, Bagdasarian A, Colman R, Nemerson Y. Activation of bovine factor VII by Hageman factor fragments. Blood 1977; 50: 611–17.
11. Jesty J, Morrison SA. The activation of factor IX by tissue factor-factor VII in a bovine plasma system lacking factor X. Thromb Res 1983; 32: 171–81.
12. Born VJJ, Reinalda-Poot JH, Cupers R, Bertina RM. Extrinsic activation of human blood coagulation factors IX and X. Thromb Haemostas 1990; 63: 224–30.
13. Rao LVM, Rapaport SI, Bajaj SP. Activation of human factor VII in the initiation of tissue factor-dependent coagulation. Blood 1986; 68: 685–91.
14. Rao LVM, Rapaport SI. Activation of factor VII bound to tissue factor: a key early step in the tissue factor pathway of blood coagulation. Proc Natl Acad Sci USA 1988; 85: 6687–91.
15. Sanders NL, Bajaj SP, Zivelin A, Rapaport SI. Inhibition of tissue factor/factor VII activity in plasma requires factor X and an additional plasma component. Blood 1985; 66: 204–12.
16. Bloom AL. Inherited disorders of blood coagulation. In: Bloom AL, Thomas DP, eds. Haemostasis and Thrombosis, 2nd ed. Edinburgh: Churchill Livingstone, 1987; 393–441.
17. Roberts HR, Foster PA. Inherited disorders of prothrombin conversion. In: Colman RW, Hirsh J, Marder VJ, Salzman EW, eds. Hemostasis and thrombosis, 2nd ed. Philadelphia: Lippincott, 1987; 162–81.
18. Meade TW, North WRS, Chakrabarti R, Stirling Y, Haines AP, Thompson SG. Haemostatic function and cardiovascular death: early results of a prospective study. Lancet 1980; 1: 1050–4.
19. Meade TW. Factor VII and ischaemic heart disease: epidemiological evidence. Haemostasis 1983; 13: 178–85.
20. Meade TW, Mellows S, Brozovic M, Miller SG, Chakrabarti RR, North WRS, Haines AP, Stirling Y, Imeson ID, Thomson SG. Haemostatic function and ischaemic heart disease: Principal results of the Northwick Park Heart Study. Lancet 1986; 2: 533–7.
21. Meade TW. The epidemiology of haemostatic and other variables in coronary artery disease. In: Verstraete M, Vermylen J, Lijnen HR, Arnout J, eds. Thrombosis and haemostasis. Leuven University Press 1987; 37–60.

22. Miller GJ, Seghatchian MJ, Walter SJ, Howarth DJ, Thompson SG, Esnouf MP, Meade TW. An association between the factor VII coagulant activity and thrombin activity induced by surface/cold exposure of normal human plasma. Br J Haematol 1986; 62: 379–84.
23. Scarabin PY, Bonithon-Kopp C, Bara L, Malmejac A, Guize L, Samama M. Factor VII activation and menopausal status. Thromb Res 1990; 57: 227–34.
24. Dalaker K, Hjermann I, Prydz H. A novel form of factor VII in plasma from men at risk for cardiovascular disease. Br J Haematol 1985; 61: 315–22.
25. Scarabin PY, Van Dreden P, Bonithon-Kop C, Orssaud G, Bara L, Conard J, Samama M. Age related changes in factor VII activation in healthy women. Clin Sci 1988; 75: 341–3.
26. Hoffman C, Shak A, Sodums M, Hultin MB. Factor VII activity state in coronary artery disease. J Lab Clin Med 1988; 111: 475–81.
27. Miller GJ, Walter SJ, Stirling Y, Thompson SG, Esnouf MP, Meade TW. Assay of factor VII activity by two techniques: evidence for increased conversion of VII to alpha VIIa in hyperlipaemia, with possible implications for ischaemic heart disease. Br J Haematol 1985; 59: 249–58.
28. Czendlik C, Lämmle B, Duckert F. Cold promoted activation and factor XII, prekallikrein and C_1-inhibitor. Thromb Haemostas 1985; 53: 242–4.
29. Gjnnaess H. Cold promoted activation of factor VII. Occurrence and relation to sex hormones and antifertility compounds. Gynaecol Invest 1973; 4: 61–72.
30. Seligsohn U, Osterud B, Brown SF, Griffin JH, Rapaport SI. Activation of human factor VII in plasma and purified systems. Roles of activated factor IX, kallikrein and activated factor XII. J Clin Invest 1979; 64: 1056–65.
31. Barrowcliffe TW, Curtis AD. Principles of bioassay. In: Bloom AL, Thomas DP, eds. Haemostasis and thrombosis. Edinburgh: Churchill Livingstone, 1987; 996–1004.
32. Finney DJ. Statistical method in biological assay, 3rd ed. London: Charles Griffin, 1978.
33. Brandt JT, Triplett DA, Fair DS. Characterization and comparison of immune-depleted and hereditary factor VII-deficient plasmas as substrate plasma for factor VII assays. Am J Clin Pathol 1986; 85: 583–9.
34. Takase T, Tuddenham EG, Chand S, Goodall AH. Monoclonal antibodies to human factor VII: production of immunodepleted plasma for VII:C assays. J Clin Pathol 1988; 41: 342–5.
35. Triplett DA, Brandt JT, Batard MA, Dixon JL, Fair DS. Hereditary factor VII deficiency, heterogeneity defined by combined functional and immunochemical analysis. Blood 1985; 66: 1284–7.
36. Bertina RM, Orlando M, Tiedemann-Aderkamp GH. Preparation of a human factor VII deficient plasma. Thromb Res 1978; 13: 537–41.
37. Mustard JF, Secord D, Hoeksema TD, Downie HG, Rowsell HC. Canine factor VII deficiency. Br J Haematol 1962; 8: 4347–54.
38. Garner R, Conning DM. The assay of human factor VII by means of modified factor VII deficient dog plasma. Br J Haematol 1970; 18: 57–66.
39. Poller L, Thomson JM, Sear CHJ, Thomas W. Identification of a congenital defect of factor VII in a colony of beagle dogs: The clinical use of the plasma. J Clin Pathol 1971; 24: 626–31.
40. Duckert F. Analytische Methoden. In: Koller F, Duckert F, eds. Thrombose und Embolie. Stuttgart: Schattauer, 1983; 761–78.
41. Thomson JM, Poller L. Factor VIII assay proficiency assessment: experience in the UK. Scand J Haematol 1984; 33 (Suppl. 41): 101–8.
42. Maas RL, Triplett DA, Tholen D. Factor VIII assay proficiency assessment: experience in the USA. Scand J Haematol 1984; 33 (Suppl. 41); 109–20.
43. Thompson SG, Duckert F, Haverkate F, Thomson JM. The measurement of haemostatic factors in the European laboratories: quality assessment for the multicentre ECAT Angina pectoris study. Thromb Haemostas 1989; 61: 301–6.
44. Seligsohn U, Osterud B, Rapaport SL. Coupled amidolytic assay for factor VII: its use with a clotting assay to determine the activity state of factor VII. Blood 1978; 52: 978–88.
45. Boyer C, Wolf M, Rothschild C, Migand M, Amiral J, Mannucci PM, Meyer D, Larrieu MJ. An enzyme immunoassay (ELISA) for the quantitation of human factor VII. Thromb Haemostas 1986; 56: 250–5.
46. Takase T, Tuddenham EG, Chand S, Goodall AH. Monoclonal antibodies to human factor VII: a one step immunoradiometric assay for VII: Ag. J Clin Pathol 1988; 41: 337–41.

47. Tirindelli MC, Mariani G, Mazzucconi MG, Iacopino G, Carbonaro M, Ghirardini A, Motta M, Mandelli F. Evaluation of factor VII antigen in factor VII congenital deficiencies with a new ELISA assay. Am J Hematol 1987; 26: 313–21.
48. Carvalho de Sousa J, Azevedo J, Soria C, Barros F, Ribeiro C, Parreira F, Caen JP. Factor VII hyperactivity in acute myocardial thrombosis. A relation to the coagulation activation. Thromb Res 1988; 51: 165–73.

8
Factor VIII clotting activity

P. M. MANNUCCI and A. TRIPODI

INTRODUCTION

Factor VIII activity has been historically measured with two types of methods: the *one-stage assay*, based on the activated partial thromboplastin time (APTT) and the *two-stage assay*, based on the thromboplastin generation test. The relative merits of the two assays have been debated[1,2]. In general, results obtained on the same samples are similar; however, discrepancies can be seen in plasmas which contain activated factors of the coagulation cascade. These factors make the clotting times obtained with the one-stage assay shorter than expected on the basis of the factor VIII content, resulting in a significant overestimation of the factor VIII activity. For the same reason the one-stage assay is often unsuitable to determine factor VIII in concentrates. Even though the two-stage assay does not seem to suffer from the same drawback, it is difficult to perform because the reagents employed need a high degree of standardization difficult to achieve in less specialized clinical laboratories.

More recently, new two-stage methods which employ chromogenic substrate have been proposed for the measurement of factor VIII[3,4]; commercial kits are available from various manufacturers (Kabi Diagnostica, Stockholm, Sweden; Baxter Dade, Miami, Florida; Diagnostica Stago, Asnieres, France) and some of them have been evaluated and found suitable for clinical application[5,6]. However, to our knowledge, their use is still limited and more extensive clinical validation is probably needed. For this reason we have chosen to discuss here the one-stage assay. More information on the other assays can be found in the cited references. Before giving details of the method we shall provide a brief account of the general principles of bioassays on which factor VIII and other clotting factor assays are based.

ASSAY CHARACTERISTICS AND PRINCIPLES

Most clotting factors can be assayed by estimating the degree of shortening of the clotting time brought about by suitable dilutions of the test plasma added to a clotting system specifically deficient in the factor to be measured. Clotting times will then be compared with those obtained when a dilution of reference plasma is added to the same system, and the activity of the unknown samples is expressed as potency relative to the reference plasma. Hence, the essential components of the bioassay are the *test system* (i.e. the clotting system) specially deficient in the factor to be assayed and the *reference plasma*. The following paragraphs outline the main components of the factor VIII clotting bioassay.

Test system

The theory of the bioassay implies that when two samples at different factor VIII activities (test and reference) are processed at different doses (dilutions) with the specific assay system (APTT), this will give different responses (clotting times). If those responses are plotted against the corresponding log-transformed factor VIII activity one should obtain a pair of dose–response curves which are parallel throughout their length. The horizontal distance between the two curves is a measure of the potency ratio between the two samples (Figure 8.1). It is important to emphasize that parallelism of the two curves is a prerequisite for correct estimation of factor VIII activity. The occurrence of substantial deviation from parallelism means that the two samples are not treated in the same way by the system. In most cases deviation from parallelism is likely to be due to the presence of an inhibitory substance in patient plasma or to the deficiency in the substrate plasma of factor(s) other than that to be measured.

This situation may occur, for instance, when substrate plasma used for the assay has lost the activity of the labile factor V during prolonged and/or poor storage conditions. To establish parallelism, patient and reference plasma must be run at several dilutions. Hence, the simplified and widely adopted procedure of testing a complete dose–response curve for reference plasma and only one dilution of the test plasma must be regarded as incorrect. As mentioned above, the system must be deficient in the factor to be measured. The most obvious and cheap solution to this problem is the plasma from a patient with severe haemophilia A (factor VIII clotting activity < 1 U/dl) with no antibody to factor VIII. This solution is, however, less and less practicable because the increasing risk of transmission of virus-related infections makes the majority of severe haemophilic patients unsuitable for the purpose. A valid alternative is to rely on factor VIII-deficient plasmas obtained by artificial depletion of normal plasma by means of monoclonal antibody against factor VIII[7]. Commercial immunodepleted plasmas are also available (e.g. Ortho Diagnostic Systems, Raritan, NJ; Diagnostica Stago).

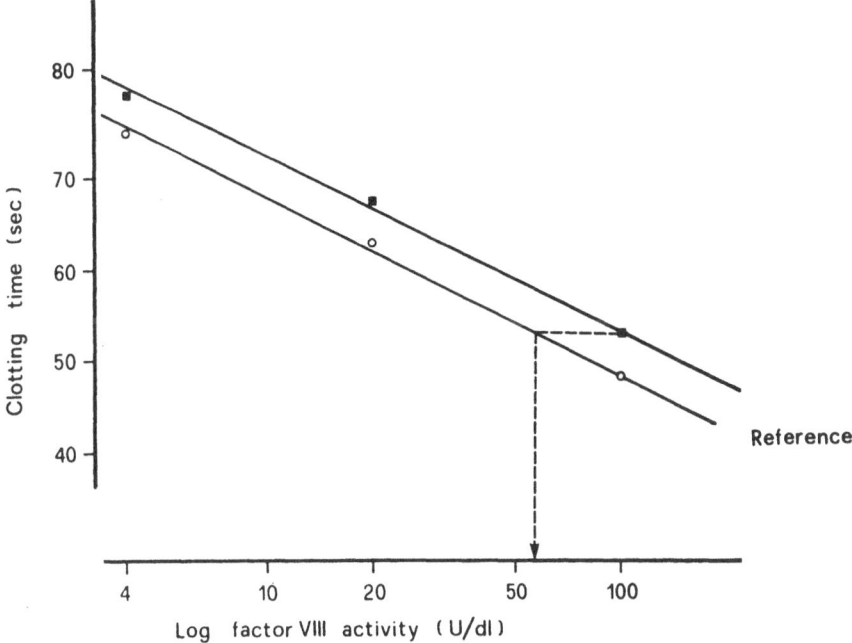

Figure 8.1 Graphical calculation of factor VIII clotting activity. The dilutions for the reference and patient plasmas were 1:10; 1:50 and 1:250. According to the graphical calculation (see text), the factor VIII activity for the patient plasma is 57 U/dl of the reference; if the potency of the reference calibrated against the international standard is 0.85 then the final result will be $57 \times 0.85 = 48$ IU/dl. Should the patient plasma be tested at higher or lower dilution than the reference, the results must be multiplied or divided by the appropriate dilution factor

Reference plasma

A convenient source of reference plasma is plasma pooled from a suitable number of healthy donors. It is important to note that plasma pooled from an insufficient number of donors might not be representative of the average value in the normal population. Hence, the assignment of an arbitrary potency of 100 U/dl may lead to important under- or overestimations of factor VIII levels in the test sample.

Due to the large biological variability in the normal population (factor VIII in normals varies from 50 to 150 U/dl), the adequacy of a pooled plasma in reflecting the average normal content of factor VIII is largely dependent on the number of healthy donors selected for the preparation. Fifty or more donors seems to be an adequate number. However, collecting such a large number of donors might be impracticable and not strictly necessary. At least in theory, plasma from a single donor is suitable as reference plasma, provided it is calibrated against the International Standard for Factor VIII/von Willebrand Factor, which is available upon request from the National Institute for Biological Standards and Control (Blanche Lane, South Mimms, Potters Bar, Hertfordshire, EN6 3QG, UK). The calibration is made by assaying the local reference plasma against the International Standard. To minimize error it is important to carry out at least four independent assays which involve a completely fresh set of the International Standard and test dilutions each time. Since the supply of Standard is often limited, a suitable alternative might be to perform two assays from the same vial of the reconstituted Standard. The potency of the local plasma is eventually obtained by multiplying the calculated potency by that of the International Standard.

METHOD

Due to the large variation in sensitivity to factor VIII among commercial APTT reagents it is impossible to give technical details which apply to all. As a general rule each laboratory should establish the best conditions with the chosen reagent. For instance, it is advisable to make a complete dose–response curve by testing several dilutions of reference plasma. The first dilution should be sufficiently high to avoid interference with other plasma components; usually a 1:5 or 1:10 dilution is suitable to start with and the other dilutions should be spaced by the same factor (i.e. for a factor of five, 1:10, 1:50, 1:250, 1:1250, etc.). It is advisable to use the same dilution interval for standard and patient plasma alike. The last dilution to be tested depends on the reagent and substrate plasma used; usually, it will be the one whose clotting time is close to, but shorter than, that of the 'blank' (i.e. sample replaced by buffer). For choosing the most suitable standard dilutions it is advisable to inspect the dose–response curve and choose at least three dilutions which lie on the steeper and linear part of the curve.

The dilutions of patient plasma should be chosen in accordance with the expected factor VIII activity. In general patient clotting times should be as close as possible to, but longer than, those of the reference plasma. Therefore if the standard is run at 1:10, 1:50, and 1:250, the patient plasma will be tested either at 1:5, 1:25 and 1:125; or 1:20, 1:100 and 1:500 when lower or higher than normal factor VIII activity is expected. To avoid the time-trend deterioration of samples and reagents, it is advisable to take replicate readings of each dilution in a balanced order (i.e. starting from the first dilution of the standard to the last of the patient samples and the replicate in the opposite order).

Estimation of the potency of a patient sample relative to the standard can be done by using a graphical or mathematical solution. The latter is preferable because it avoids bias in fitting the dose–response curves and gives objective criteria to assess for linearity and parallelism. Simple calculations can be performed by pocket calculator, as described by Ingram[8]. Comprehensive statistical advice on writing computer programs for bioassay are beyond the scope of this chapter, and can be found in the published literature[9–11]. For the graphical calculation, the mean values of the replicate readings for each dilution are plotted (vertical axis) against the log-transformed percentage activity (horizontal axis), the first dilution of the reference and patient plasmas being arbitrarily taken as 100 U/dl activity (Figure 8.1). After drawing the best-fit lines through the data points and checking for parallelism, the activity of factor VIII in patient plasma is derived by drawing a horizontal line from the point where the patient curve intercepts the 100 U/dl activity to the point where it crosses the reference curve. From that point a vertical line is then dropped to intercept the horizontal axis. This value represents the percentage activity of factor VIII in the patient plasma relative to the reference (Figure 8.1). When patient plasma is tested at a higher or lower dilution than the standard, the result must be multiplied or divided by the appropriate dilution factor.

The procedure outlined below is intended to fit the characteristics of the commercial APTT reagent and coagulometer currently used in our laboratory. Other preparations can be successfully used provided the optimal conditions are chosen as recommended above.

Reagents

1. Automated APTT (Organon Teknika, Durham, NC). This reagent contains micronized silica as activator and rabbit brain phospholipids as platelet substitute.
2. Imidazole buffer is prepared by dissolving 3.4 g of imidazole and 5.85 g NaCl in approximately 70 ml distilled water; 18.6 ml of 1 mmol/L HCl is then added, the pH adjusted to 7.3–7.4 and the final volume adjusted to 100 ml. This stock solution is stored at 4 °C and used to prepare the working solution by diluting it 1:10 with distilled water.
3. $CaCl_2$, 0.025 mol/L.
4. Substrate plasma with factor VIII content < 1 U/dl.
5. Reference plasma calibrated against the International Standard for Factor VIII/von Willebrand Factor.

Equipment

1. Plastic tubes to make dilutions.
2. Automated micropipettes equipped with plastic tips.
3. Photo-optical or mechanical coagulometer (Coag A Mate X 2, Organon Teknika, or other commercial brand). The procedure described can also be carried out with the manual tilt-tube technique.

Procedure

1. Three dilutions (1:10, 1:50 and 1:250) of the reference and patient plasma should be prepared immediately before starting the assay. As mentioned above, the actual dilution of patient plasma will depend on the expected factor VIII activity, a rough idea thereof being obtained by the APTT value of the test plasma.
2. One hundred microlitres of each dilution is pipetted into the wells of the coagulometer in balanced order (see above).
3. Add 100 µl of substrate plasma.
4. Pipette (or program the coagulometer to do so) 100 µl APTT reagent.

5. Incubate the mixture for exactly 5 min (if other reagent is used, follow the instructions of the manufacturer).
6. At the end of the incubation add 100 µl $CaCl_2$, 0.025 mol/L.
7. Record the clotting time which will be used for the calculation of factor VIII activity (see above).

NORMAL VALUES

Factor VIII clotting activity in the normal population varies between 50 and 150 U/dl; it is recommended that each laboratory establish its own normal range.

CLINICAL RELEVANCE OF FACTOR VIII MEASUREMENT

The measurement of factor VIII clotting activity in plasma is essential in diagnosing patients with haemophilia A and monitoring their treatment with factor VIII concentrates. Low levels of factor VIII are also found in patients with acquired antibodies to factor VIII and in disseminated intravascular coagulation. Factor VIII activity is increased transiently after beta-adrenoreceptor stimulation such as physical exercise and emotional stress, and after infusion of pharmacological agents such as desmopressin (DDAVP). Since factor VIII is an acute-phase reactant, long-term increases can be expected during inflammatory diseases and in post-surgical patients.

References

1. Kirkwood TBL, Rizza CR, Snape TJ, Rhymes IL, Austen DEG. Identification of sources of interlaboratory variation in factor VIII assay. Br J Haematol 1981; 37: 559–68.
2. Nilsson IM, Kirkwood TBL, Barrowcliffe TW. In vivo recovery of factor VIII: comparison of one-stage and two-stage assay methods. Thromb Haemostas 1979; 42: 1230–9.
3. Segatchian MJ, Miller-Andersson M. A colorimetric evalution of factor VIII:C. Med Lab Sci 1978; 35: 347–54.
4. Rosen S, Andersson M, Mikaelsson M, Oswaldsson U. Determination of factor VIII activity with chromogenic substrate kit method. I. Basic performance. Thromb Haemostas 1984; 40: 139–45.
5. Rosen S, Andersson M, Blomback M et al. Clinical application of a chromogenic substrate method for the determination of factor VIII activity. Thromb Haemostas 1985; 54: 818–23.
6. Tripodi A, Mannucci PM. Factor VIII activity as measured by an amidolytic assay compared with a one-stage clotting assay. Am J Clin Pathol 1986; 86: 341–4.
7. Takase T, Rotblat F, Goodall AH, Kernoff PBA, Middleton S, Chand S, Denson KW, Austen DEG, Tuddenham EGD. Production of factor VIII deficient plasma by immunodepletion using three monoclonal antibodies. Br J Haematol 1987; 66: 497–502.
8. Ingram GIC. Blood coagulation factor VIII: genetics, physiological control and bioassay. In: Sobotka H, Stewart CP, eds. Advances in clinical chemistry, vol. 8. New York: Academic Press, 1965; 189–236.
9. Counts RB, Hayes JE. A computer program for analysis of clotting factor assays and other parallel-line bioassay. Am J Clin Pathol 1979; 71: 167–71.
10. Williams KN, Davidson JMF, Ingram GIC. A computer program for the analysis of parallel-line bioassays of clotting factors. Br J Haematol 1975; 31: 13–23.
11. Kirkwood TBL, Snape TJ. Biometric principles in clotting and clot lysis assays. Clin Lab Haematol 1980; 2: 155–67.

9
Von Willebrand factor

P. M. MANNUCCI and R. COPPOLA

INTRODUCTION

Human von Willebrand factor (vWF) can be measured by functional and immunological assays. *Functional assays* explore the ability of plasma vWF to agglutinate platelets in the presence of the antibiotic ristocetin; hence, this method is known as ristocetin cofactor activity assay[1]. The measurement of ristocetin cofactor activity is complicated by the need to prepare a standardized suspension of formaldehyde-fixed normal platelets, which makes the assay unsuitable for less specialized laboratories. The *immunological assays* are based on the electroimmunoassay (EIA) of patient and standard samples in agarose-containing rabbit antibodies to human vWF[2,3]. At optimal conditions of pH and ionic strength the antigen–antibody complexes precipitate as narrow rocket-shaped peaks which allow the quantitation of vWF antigen by comparing the peak heights of the patient samples with those of standards containing known amounts of vWF. More recently, methods based on enzyme-linked immunosorbent assay (ELISA) have been proposed for the measurement of vWF[4,5], with commercial kits available from several manufacturers (e.g. Diagnostica Stago, Asnieres, France; American Diagnostica, New York). In general, results obtained with the EIA are in close agreement with those obtained with ELISA. However, better precision, together with higher sensitivity, makes ELISA the method of choice for vWF antigen measurement.

PRINCIPLES AND ASSAY CHARACTERISTICS

The method is based on the sandwich principle. In the first step, plastic wells of microtitre plates are coated with antibodies against vWF (capture antibody). In the second step, suitable dilutions of test and standard plasmas are incubated to allow vWF antigen to bind the capture antibody. After washing the wells to remove the unbound antigen, a second antibody to vWF labelled with horseradish peroxidase (detecting antibody) is added. This results in the formation of a sandwich complex in a quantity proportional to the vWF content in patient and standard plasmas. After a second washing to remove excess detecting antibody, the peroxidase activity is measured photometrically by addition of hydrogen peroxide and O-phenylenediamine. The optical density readings are then converted into U/dl of vWF antigen by comparison with a calibration curve obtained by processing dilutions of a pooled normal plasma or standard plasma.

METHOD

Recently we produced and characterized five murine monoclonal antibodies (MoAb) to human vWF. All MoAbs were positive in a direct ELISA and in multimeric analysis of purified vWF; competition experiments set up after conjugation of peroxidase showed that two of them (11B6.18 and 7G10.8) were directed against different vWF epitopes and were therefore used as capture and detecting antibodies to set up an ELISA assay for measuring vWF antigen[6]. This method may be used as a guideline to set up methods with home made or commercial antibodies to vWF.

Reagents

1. Coating buffer: 50 mmol/L Tris-HCl, pH 9.00.
2. Over-coating buffer: as for coating buffer, added with 3% bovine serum albumin.
3. Washing buffer: 20 mmol/L Tris-HCl, 100 mmol/L NaCl, 0.1% Tween, 0.1% bovine serum albumin, pH 7.4.
4. Dilution buffer: as for washing buffer, with added 0.5% bovine serum albumin.
5. Substrate buffer: 22 mmol/L trisodium citrate, 50 mmol/L Na_2HPO_4. Adjust pH to 5.5 with H_3PO_4.
6. 400 µg/ml o-phenylenediamine (Sigma, St Louis, MO).
7. 30% H_2O_2.
8. 3 mol/L H_2SO_4.
9. Two different monoclonal antibodies were used as capture and detecting antibodies.

Immediately before use, prepare a solution of o-phenylenediamine 40 mg and H_2O_2 40 µl and make the volume to 100 ml with substrate buffer.

Procedure

The detecting antibody was conjugated with horseradish peroxidase (Sigma) (final concentration 250 µg/ml) according to the method of Nakane and Kawaoi[7] and stored in small aliquots at $-20\,°C$ in the presence of glycerol

(50% final concentration). Polystyrene plates (Nunc, Roskilde, Denmark) are coated overnight at 4 °C with 125 µl/well of a 2.5 µg/ml solution of capture antibody in coating buffer. At the end of the incubation the solution is discarded and the wells are overcoated with 200 µl of over-coating buffer for 1 or 2 h. The wells are then washed three times with washing buffer and added with 100 µl/well of standard plasma (in duplicate) diluted from 1:50 to 1:3200 in dilution buffer. Patient samples are tested at two different dilutions chosen according to the expected concentration of vWF in the sample (usually, 1:100 and 1:400). After incubation for 2 h (or overnight) at room temperature, the wells are washed three times and added with 100 µl/well of detecting antibody (5 µg/ml) in dilution buffer. After incubation for 1 h at room temperature, the wells are washed three times and added with 100 µl/well of o-phenylenediamine and H_2O_2 solution. After incubation for 10 min at room temperature (dark), the reaction is stopped by adding 50 µl/well H_2SO_4. The optical density is then measured at 486 nm with a microplate photometer. vWF antigen in patient samples is derived by extrapolation from the calibration curve (Figure 9.1).

Results obtained with the above method in plasma samples from healthy subjects and patients with von Willebrand disease compared favourably with those obtained with the commercial kit Asserachrom vWF (Diagnostica Stago Asnieres, France), which can be used as a suitable alternative.

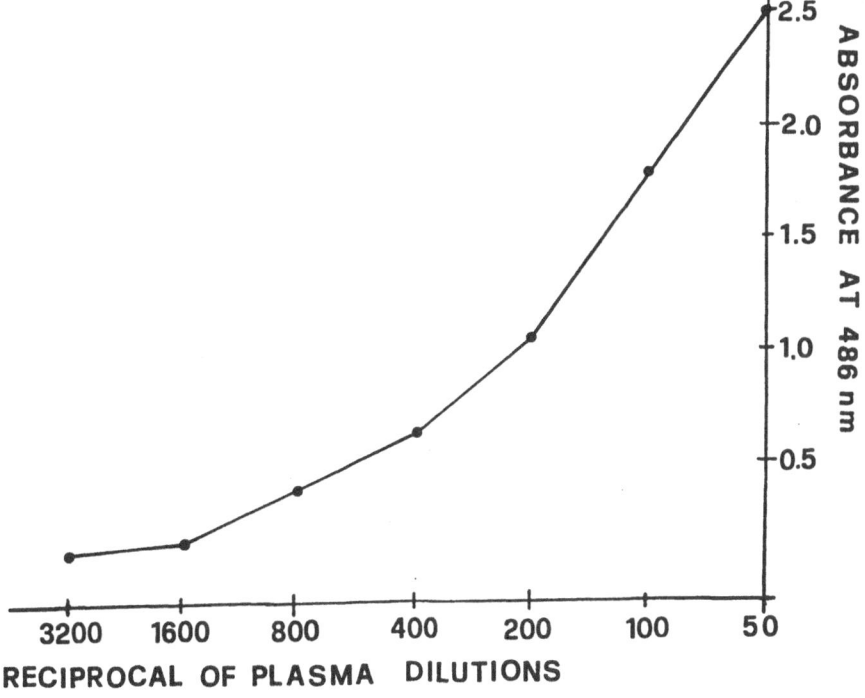

Figure 9.1 Plasma dilution curve of vWF antigen in pooled normal plasma

REFERENCE PLASMA

As mentioned for factor VIII clotting assay, plasmas from a large number of healthy donors must be pooled in order to get a standard truly representative of the average normal plasma and hence suitable to construct the calibration curve for vWF antigen assay. Fifty or more healthy donors, equally divided between males and females and covering different age classes, are adequate. As an alternative a pooled plasma from a limited number of donors (even from a single donor) can be used, provided such plasma is first calibrated against the International Standard for factor VIII and vWF (National Institute for Biological Standards and Control, Blanche Lane, South Mimms, Potters Bar, Hertfordshire, EN6 3QG, UK). For details on the calibration procedure, see Chapter 8.

NORMAL RANGE

vWF antigen in the normal population varies between 50 and 150 U/dl. However, age group- and blood group-related differences have been reported within the same population[8,9]. In general, vWF antigen increases with increasing age and blood group O values are on average lower than those of non-group O. Accordingly, it is strongly recommended that each laboratory establish its own normal range.

CLINICAL SIGNIFICANCE OF vWF ANTIGEN MEASUREMENT

The measurement of plasma vWF antigen is essential to differentiate between haemophilia A and von Willebrand's disease. In haemophilia vWF antigen is normal, whereas factor VIII is low. In von Willebrand's disease vWF antigen is usually low, being moderately reduced in type I and severely reduced in type III. However, a normal level of vWF antigen does not exclude the diagnosis of von Willebrand's disease, because molecular variants of the disease have normal or near-normal vWF antigen and reduced ristocetin cofactor activity (type II) (for a comprehensive review of vWF classification see ref. 10). Being an acute-phase reactant, vWF is increased during inflammatory diseases and in postsurgical patients. In addition, a number of other clinical conditions such as diabetes mellitus, atherosclerosis, liver cirrhosis, tumours, uraemia, pregnancy-induced hypertension and thrombocytopenic purpura have been described in which plasma vWF antigen levels are increased.

References

1. MacFarlane DE, Stibbe J, Kirby EP, Zucker MB, Grant RA, McPherson J. A method for assaying von Willebrand factor (ristocetin cofactor). Thromb Diath Haemorrh 1975; 34: 306–8.
2. Laurell CB. Quantitative estimation of proteins by electrophoresis in agarose gel containing antibodies. Anal Biochem 1966; 15: 45–52.

3. Zimmerman TS, Hoyer LW, Dickson L, Edgington TS. Determination of the von Willebrand's disease antigen (factor VIII related antigen) in plasma by quantitative immunoelectrophoresis. J Lab Clin Med 1975; 86: 152–9.
4. Bartlett A, Dormandy KM, Hawkey CM, Stableforth P, Voller A. Factor VIII-related antigen: measurement by enzyme immunoassay. Br Med J 1976; 1: 994–6.
5. Silveira AMV, Yamamoto T, Adamson L, Hessel B, Blomback B. Application of an enzyme-linked immunosorbent assay (ELISA) to von Willebrand factor (vWF) and its derivatives. Thromb Res 1986; 43: 91–102.
6. Federici AB, Tombesi S, Coppola R, Colibretti ML, Gobbi A, Albertini A, Mannucci PM. Preliminary results on the characterization of monoclonal antibodies to von Willebrand factor (vWF). Abstract of the International Symposium on Biotechnology of plasma proteins: Haemostasis, thrombosis and iron proteins. Florence, 9–11 April, 1990.
7. Nakane PK, Kawaoi PA. Peroxidase-labeled antibody: a new method of conjugation. J Histochem Cytochem 1974; 22: 1084–91.
8. Cox Gill J, Endres-Brooks J, Bauer PJ, Marks WJ, Montgomery RR. The effect of ABO blood group on the diagnosis of von Willebrand disease. Blood 1987; 69: 1691–5.
9. Rodeghiero F, Castaman G, Dini E. Epidemiological investigation of the prevalence of von Willebrand's disease. Blood 1987; 69: 454–9.
10. Ruggeri ZM, Zimmerman TS. von Willebrand factor and von Willebrand disease. Blood 1987; 74: 895–904.

10
Antithrombin III activity and antigen

J. CONARD

INTRODUCTION

Antithrombin III (AT III) is a major physiological inhibitor of blood coagulation. It inactivates mainly thrombin, but also activated factors X, IX, XI and XII. Heparin accelerates the reaction between AT III and heparin, and this explains why AT III is also called 'Heparin cofactor'[1,2].

AT III is important in maintaining haemostatic balance, as demonstrated by the increased risk of thrombosis observed in patients with congenital deficiency. It can be measured by different methods: immunological or functional, and quantitative as well as qualitative deficiencies have been reported.

SAMPLING AND STORAGE

Citrated blood is commonly used: sodium citrate 0.11 mol/L (1 volume) and blood (9 volumes). The anticoagulated blood is centrifuged at 2000 g or more for 20 min. At least 0.5 ml of plasma is transferred to small plastic tubes that are stoppered and kept in a freezer at −20 °C or lower. They can be stored up to 4 months before assay.

At the time of the test, samples are rapidly thawed at 37 °C. Lipaemic plasmas may not be suitable for nephelometric assays.

STANDARD AND CONTROLS

1. AT III standard: a freeze-dried AT III standard can be obtained from the National Institute for Biological Standards and Control, Blanche Lane, South Mimms, Potters Bar, Herts EN6 3QG, UK.
2. Local reference plasma: the local reference plasma is prepared from a mixture of equal amounts of citrated plasmas from more than 20 healthy

77

individuals of both sexes, taking no oral contraceptive or other medication. Aliquots are frozen at $-20\,°C$ or lower.
3. AT III control plasmas: different control plasmas (normal or pathological range) are commercially available, from Kabi, Behringwerke, Ortho or Stago, for instance.

ACTIVITY ASSAYS[3-5]

AT III may be measured: (a) by clotting or chromogenic method: the latter is the most commonly used because the clotting method requires defibrination of the plasma and is more difficult to standardize; (b) in the presence (heparin cofactor activity) or the absence of heparin (progressive antithrombin activity). Heparin cofactor activity is preferred in routine practice because it allows the detection of all types of AT III deficiencies, quantitative as well as functional (type I and II).

The chromogenic method for heparin cofactor activity may be done using commercially available kits and will be described here.

Principle

Plasma AT III is determined as the capacity for inactivating thrombin in the presence of heparin. Heparin has a catalytic effect on the reaction AT III – thrombin. An excess of purified thrombin is added to the plasma and the amount of thrombin inactivated by the complex AT III–heparin depends on the amount of plasma AT III. Residual thrombin hydrolyses paranitroaniline (pNA) of the substrate and released pNA is measured at 405 nm. The method can be summarized as follows:

1. AT III + heparin (excess)→[AT III–heparin]
2. [AT III–heparin] + bovine thrombin (excess)→[AT III–heparin–thrombin] + thrombin (residual)
3. Substrate + residual thrombin→pNA (405 nm)

Commonly used substrates are S-2238 Kabi and CBS 3447 Stago.

Assay procedure

Endpoint assay by manual methods may be used, but kinetic automated assays are preferred for better reliability[6,7]. The following instruments are suitable: Cobas Bio, Chromotimer Behringwerke, Gilford, Hitachi, etc.

Bovine thrombin seems more appropriate than human thrombin in order to avoid the interference of heparin cofactor II[8,9].

Special case: ACA Du Pont method

The ACA method is a 'closed' system requiring ACA SX Instrument and packs. The principle is as follows:

1. AT III + bovine thrombin (excess) + heparin (excess)→[thrombin–AT III] + thrombin (residual)
2. Z-Lys–SBzl + residual thrombin→Z-Lys + SBzl
3. SBzl + DTNB→chromophore (452 nm)

The residual thrombin catalyses the hydrolysis of α-N-carbobenzyloxy-L-lysine thiobenzylester (Z-Lys-SBzl). The hydrolysis product, α-toluenethiol (SBzl) further reacts with DTNB [5,5'-dithiobis-(2-nitrobenzoic acid)] to form the chromophore.

The calibration of the AT III assay may be performed using the lyophilized controls from ACA, but we prefer to use our local reference pool plasma obtained from more than 20 healthy subjects, as mentioned above. The local reference plasma is checked undiluted (100%), 1:1 (50%) and 1:2 (33%). Once the calibration is performed for a batch of AT III reagents packs it is remarkably stable; however, it is recommended to control it twice a month and to test pathological and normal lyophilized control plasmas regularly.

ANTIGEN ASSAYS

AT III may be measured immunologically by radial immunodiffusion, electroimmunodiffusion or laser nephelometry[10]. In the previous ECAT Book the Laurell method was recommended, but we will describe here the nephelometric assay with Behring instrument and reagents, because we use it routinely.

Principle

Immunoprecipitation is performed in a liquid phase by adsorption on latex particules. A laser nephelometer measures light scattered in a forward direction by immunocomplexes in an incident beam of monochromatic light. The diffuse light is measured in an angle between 13° and 24°. The reading is performed at 840 nm.

Instrument

The Behring Nephelometer Analyser (BNA) is an automated instrument, convenient to perform large series of AT III determinations (45 cuvettes divided into nine segments of five cuvettes each).

Reagents and standard

AT III antiserum and a normal plasma protein standard are provided by Behringwerke. Results of the standard are expressed in mg/dl and are usually 30 mg/ml, but we prefer to give the results as a percentage of the local normal pool.

Assay procedure

After the plasmas have been introduced into the cuvettes all steps are automatic. If the result is marked with a cross it may be incorrect because the plasma is lipaemic: centrifugation may help in this respect. Haemolysis does not interfere.

NORMAL VALUES

Normal values are in the range 80–120%.

AT III levels are reduced in some physiological conditions such as the neonatal period[11,12]. In men AT III tends to decrease after the age of 50, while in women a menopausal influence has been suspected to explain the observed increase[13,14]. During normal pregnancy, AT III may slightly decrease but usually remains in the normal range[15].

CONGENITAL DEFICIENCY IN AT III[16–18]

Congenital AT III deficiency is classically associated with a high risk of thrombosis. It is considered as a rare finding: 2–4% in patients with history of venous thromboembolism. The deficiency is transmitted as an autosomal dominant trait.

The first episode is usually observed between the ages of 20 and 30, and about 85% of the patients older than 50 have had at least one thrombosis. A triggering factor (pregnancy, oral contraceptive, surgical procedure, immobilization) is often present, but no known predisposition factor is found in approximately half the cases.

Heterozygous affected members have a level of about 50–60% of the normal value. Comparison of the levels of heparin cofactor activity and antigen level allows the detection of different types of AT III deficiencies[19]:

1. Type I characterized by a parallel decrease of AT III activity and antigen. Subtypes Ia: reduced synthesis and/or increased turnover of a normal molecule; Ib: reduced synthesis and/or turnover of antithrombin with abnormal heparin binding.
2. Type II with a normal antigen level associated with a decreased AT III activity. Subtypes IIa: functional abnormalities affecting both the reactive site and heparin binding site; IIb: functional abnormalities limited to the reactive site; IIc: functional abnormalities limited to the heparin binding site.

Subtypes of Type I and II all have decreased heparin cofactor activity; they differ by the level of AT III progressive activity (in the absence of heparin) and by the electrophoretic pattern in the presence (or absence) of heparin (Table 10.1). In normal plasma samples, crossed immunoelectrophoresis shows one peak in the presence and absence of heparin. Distinction between reactive site and heparin binding site variants is made by crossed immunoelectrophoresis in the presence of heparin: an additional cathodal

Table 10.1 Classifiction of hereditary antithrombin III deficiency

Type	Antigen	Heparin cofactor activity	Progressive activity	Heparin affinity*
Ia	↓	↓	↓	Normal
Ib	↓	↓	↓	Decreased
IIa	Normal	↓	↓	Decreased
IIb	Normal	↓	↓	Normal or increased
IIc†	Normal	↓	Normal	Decreased

* Evaluated by crossed immunoelectrophoresis
† In type IIc the risk of thrombosis is very low in heterozygous patients, in contrast with other types

peak, preceding the normal one (reduced mobility caused by abnormal reaction with heparin), is observed when a molecule has decreased heparin affinity; in contrast, only the normal peak is observed in reactive site variants.

The nature of the defect is confirmed by functional studies following purification from plasma and also after genetic studies. Different mutations located near the reactive site (Arg-393) or the heparin binding site (Arg-47, Pro-41) have been identified in AT III variants[17].

In Type IIc, where the only anomaly is a decreased level in the presence of heparin, heterozygous patients have a low risk of thrombosis and the existence of a small number of cases of homozygotes of this type suggests a different mode of inheritance[20]. Recent reports have shown that, in the normal population, the prevalence of type IIc is about 1 in 350 while the prevalence of type I is 1 in 4200[19].

Thromboses are treated by heparin alone or heparin associated with AT III concentrates, taking into account that the half-life of AT III is 2.8 days in normal conditions[21].

Some problems are at present unsolved: management of asymptomatic patients, duration of anticoagulant treatment after a thrombosis and treatment to be administered during pregnancy, since there is a high frequency of thromboses related to pregnancy[22].

ACQUIRED DEFICIENCY

Acquired deficiencies may be related to diseases or to treatments, and are inconstantly associated with thrombosis[16].

Pathological conditions

1. Liver cirrhosis: AT III is decreased in liver cirrhosis, as well as other coagulation factors and inhibitors synthesized in the liver. This deficiency is not usually associated with thrombosis.
2. Nephrotic syndrome: when the urinary loss of AT III exceeds its synthesis, a plasma deficiency is observed and may be responsible for venous thrombosis.

3. Postoperative period: a decrease has been reported after knee surgery, and since this type of surgery is highly thrombogenic it has been proposed to administer AT III concentrates in association with heparin.
4. Disseminated intravascular coagulation (DIC): AT III is inconstantly decreased and it cannot be used as a criterion for the diagnosis of DIC. It is more frequent in patients suffering from cancer with liver metastasis and also in septicaemia.

Table 10.2 Acquired deficiencies in AT III

Pathological conditions
   Liver cirrhosis
   Nephrotic syndrome
   Postoperative period
   Disseminated intravascular coagulation

Treatments
   Heparin
   Hormones
   L-Asparaginase

Treatment

1. Heparin: unfractionated heparin increases the turnover of AT III resulting in a decrease in plasma AT III. Low molecular heparins do not seem to have such an effect.
2. Hormones: oestro-progestogens induce a moderate decrease (approximately 10%) that is related to the dose of oestrogen and probably contributes to the increased risk of venous thrombosis reported during these treatments. Some progestogens, such as lynestrenol, are also responsible for a low AT III level[23]. In contrast, the natural oestrogen, 17β-oestradiol, used for replacement therapy in menopausal women, has no effect on AT III when administered by percutaneous route[24,25].
3. L-Asparaginase: this drug, used in the treatment of leukaemias and different hematological diseases, decreases AT III levels and may contribute to thromboses observed during these treatments.

CONCLUSION

The detection of congenital deficiency in AT III is of great importance since this disease is often associated with a high frequency of thrombosis and since heparin is less efficacious in these patients and AT III concentrates may be needed. However, due to the relatively high frequency of type IIc deficiencies in the normal population, and to the low or absent risk of thrombosis in these variants, it is recommended to perform the test in priority in patients with personal, and eventually family, history of thrombosis at a young age.

The method of choice for the screening is the determination of the heparin cofactor activity, because it allows the detection of all types of deficiencies.

When a deficiency is detected it is then necessary to perform the antigen assay and to classify the deficiency.

References

1. Abildgaard U. Antithrombin and related inhibitors of coagulation. In: Poller L, ed. Recent Advances in blood coagulation. Edinburgh, London, Melbourne and New York: Churchill Livingstone, 1981; 151.
2. Rosenberg RD. Action and interaction of antithrombin and heparin. N Engl J Med 1975; 16: 146–51.
3. Abildgaard U, Lie M, Ødegard OR. Antithrombin (heparin cofactor) assay with new chromogenic substrates. Thromb Res 1977; 11: 549.
4. Handeland GF, Abildgaard U, Aasen AO. Simplified assay for antithrombin III activity using chromogenic peptide substrate. Manual and automated method. Scand J Haematol 1983; 31: 427–36.
5. Ødegard OR, Abildgaard U. Antithrombin III: critical review of assay methods. Signification of variations in health and disease. Haemostasis 1978; 7: 127–34.
6. Conard J. Automation of antithrombin III. Methods on routinely available instruments. Sem Thromb Hemostas 1983; 9: 263–7.
7. Ødegard OR, Rosenlund B, Ervik E. Automated antithrombin III assay with a centrifugal analyzer. Haemostasis 1978; 7: 202–9.
8. Conard J, Horellou MH, Bara L. Bovine or human thrombin in antithrombin III (AT III) amidolytic assays. Thromb Haemostas 1985; 54: 25.
9. Friberger P, Egeberg N, Holmer E, Hellgren M, Blombäck M. Antithrombin assay. The use of human or bovine thrombin and the observation of a 'second heparin cofactor'. Thromb Res 1982; 25: 433–6.
10. Parvez Z, Fareed J, Argawal P, Messmore HI, Moncada R. Laser nephelometric quantitation of antithrombin III (AT III). Thromb Res 1981; 24: 367–77.
11. Peters M, Jansen E, Ten Cate JW, Kahlé LH, Ockelford P, Breederveld C. Neonatal antithrombin III. Br J Haematol 1984; 58: 579–87.
12. Teger-Nilsson AC. Antithrombin in infancy and childhood. Acta Paediatr Scand 1975; 64: 624–8.
13. Meade TW, Dyer S, Howarth DJ, Imeson JD, Stirling Y. Antithrombin III and procoagulant activity: sex differences and effects of the menopause. Br J Haematol 1990; 74: 77–81.
14. Tait RC, Walker ID, Davidson JF, Islam SIA, Mitchell R. Antithrombin III activity in healthy blood donors: age and sex related changes and the prevalence of asymptomatic deficiency. Br J Haematol 1990; 75: 141–2.
15. Weenink GH, Treffers PE, Kahlé LH, Ten Cate JW. Antithrombin III in normal pregnancy. Thromb Res 1982; 26: 281–7.
16. Beresford CH. Antithrombin III deficiency: Blood Rev 1988; 2: 239–50.
17. Lane DA, Caso R. Antithrombin: structure, genomic organization, function and inherited deficiency. Baillère's Clin Haematol 1989; 2: 961–98.
18. Thaler E, Lechner K. Antithrombin deficiency and thromboembolism. In: Prentice CRM, ed. Clinics in haematology. London: WB Saunders, 1981; 369–90.
19. Sas G. Hereditary antithrombin III deficiency: biochemical aspects. Haematologia (Budapest) 1984; 17: 81–6.
20. Finazzi G, Caccia R, Barbui T. Different prevalence of thromboembolism in the subtypes of congenital antithrombin III deficiency: review of 404 cases. Thrombos Haemostas 1987; 58: 1094.
21. Collen D, Schetz J, De Cock F, Holmer E, Verstraete M. Metabolism of antithrombin III in man: effects of venous thrombosis and of heparin administration. Eur J Clin Invest 1978; 7: 27–35.
22. Conard J, Horellou MH, Van Dreden P, Lecompte T, Samama M. Thrombosis and pregnancy in congenital deficiencies in AT III, protein C or protein S: study of 78 women. Thromb Haemostas 1990; 63: 319–20.
23. Bounameaux H, Duckert F, Walter M, Bounameaux Y. The determination of antithrombin III. Comparison of six methods. Effect of oral contraceptive therapy. Thromb Haemostas 1978; 39: 607–15.

24. Alkjaersig N, Fletvher AP, De Ziegler D, Steingold KA, Meldrum DR, Judd HL. Blood coagulation in postmenopausal women given estrogen treatment: comparison of transdermal and oral administration. J Lab Clin Med 1988; 111: 224–8.
25. Conard J, Samama M, Basdevant A, Guy-Grand B, De Lignières B. Differential AT III response to oral and parenteral administration of 17 β-estradiol. Thromb Haemostas 1983; 49: 252.

11
Protein C activity and antigen

R. M. BERTINA

INTRODUCTION

Protein C(PC) is a vitamin K-dependent plasma glycoprotein (MW 62 000)[1,2]. In the blood it circulates as the inactive zymogen of a serine protease (activated protein C, APC), mostly in the form of a two-chain molecule consisting of a light chain and heavy chain linked by one disulphide bond. Protein C is synthesized in the liver. During post-translational modification nine glutamic acid residues in the aminoterminus of the light chain are carboxylated by a vitamin K-dependent carboxylase. The biological half-life of protein C is about 8 h[3]. In pooled normal plasma the concentration of protein C is ~4 µg/ml (~63 nmol/L).

Physiological role

Activated protein C is the key enzyme of the protein C anticoagulant pathway. Its anticoagulant properties reside in its capacity to inactivate the cofactors Va and VIIIa by proteolytic degradation[4]. Protein S – another vitamin K-dependent plasma protein, anionic phospholipid membranes and Ca^{2+} ions are essential cofactors for the inactivation reaction[5]. By inactivating the cofactors Va and VIIIa[6,7], activated protein C will dramatically reduce the rate of thrombin formation, as can be visualized by the increase in the activated partial thromboplastin time (APTT) after addition of APC to pooled normal plasma.

The activation of protein C occurs at the endothelial surface by the thrombin–thrombomodulin complex[8]. Thrombomodulin is a membrane protein which serves as a receptor/cofactor for thrombin. Binding of thrombin to thrombomodulin changes the enzymatic properties of thrombin from a procoagulant enzyme (activation of fibrinogen and platelets) to an anticoagulant enzyme (activation of protein C). During activation an Arg–Leu bond is cleaved, after which an aminoterminal peptide of 12 amino acids is released from the heavy chain.

Under physiological conditions (i.e. in the presence of Ca^{2+}) the activation reaction is completely dependent on the availability of thrombomodulin[9]. *In vitro* protein C can be activated by thrombin in the absence of Ca^{2+} ions. However, rather high enzyme/substrate ratios are required to reach complete conversion to APC within a reasonable time interval[9].

In citrated plasma APC is neutralized by forming complexes with the APC inhibitor (PCI or PAI-3) and α_1-antitrypsin[10,11]. The reaction of APC with the APC inhibitor is accelerated to some extent by relatively high concentrations of heparin. In whole blood – that still contains physiological Ca^{2+} concentrations – APC is also neutralized by α_2-macroglobulin[12].

Pathophysiological aspects

Hereditary defects

The importance of the protein C anticoagulant system for the control of thrombin formation *in vivo* is most dramatically demonstrated in neonates who are homozygotes or double heterozygotes for hereditary protein C deficiency[13,14]. These patients develop massive and fatal (if untreated) thromboembolism shortly after birth. The most prominent clinical manifestations are large purpuric skin lesions (purpura fulminans syndrome), CNS thrombosis and central ophthalmic thrombosis.

Interestingly the clinical phenotype of heterozygotes for a hereditary protein C deficiency is not uniform. Two different phenotypes can be recognized. In the clinically dominant type of protein C deficiency heterozygotes have an increased risk of developing venous thrombosis[15–17]. Families with this type of protein C deficiency are identified by screening symptomatic patients with unexplained familial thrombophilia: about 5% of these patients are protein C-deficient[18,19]. The prevalence of this phenotype in the general population has been estimated[19] to be 1/16 000.

In the clinically recessive type of PC deficiency heterozygotes only very rarely have thrombosis[20]. Families with this type of protein C deficiency are found among the parents of homozygous protein C-deficient patients but also among healthy blood donors[13,20,21]. The prevalence of this phenotype in the general population has been estimated[21] to be 1/300.

The laboratory diagnosis of hereditary protein C deficiency focuses on the identification of homozygotes/double heterozygotes and heterozygotes of the clinically dominant form of the disorder. If not on oral anticoagulant treatment protein C (activity or antigen) levels should be lower than the lower limit of the normal range, while the plasma concentration of other vitamin K-dependent proteins is within the normal range[15,16]. The treatment of patients with oral anticoagulants offers a special problem for laboratory diagnosis because the treatment in itself causes a decrease in plasma protein C level (dependent on the intensity of the treatment). For typical therapeutic doses of coumarins protein C antigen and activity decrease to about 50% and 25%, respectively[15,22].

Therefore, in these patients protein C levels should be below the lower limit of the range observed at the relevant intensity of treatment while the ratios PC/FII, PC/FX and/or PC/FVII should also be lower than normally observed in these patients[15].

Acquired abnormalities

During the past 10 years abnormal protein C levels have been reported in a variety of clinical conditions[23]. Increased protein C levels have been reported for users of oral contraceptives[24], for patients with (acute) angina pectoris[25], and patients with a nephrotic syndrome[26,27]. Reduced levels of protein C have been reported for patients in the postoperative period[28] and for patients with liver disease[29], various forms of DIC[30], insulin-dependent diabetes[31,32], essential hypertension[33] and sickle cell disease[34]. Sometimes only a decrease in specific activity or PC activity/PC antigen ratio is observed[30]. In general it is not clear whether the reduced PC levels trigger or provoke the development of thrombosis in such patients.

Further it is important to realize that protein C levels increase with age (about 4% per decade)[35] and that treatment protocols might also influence protein C levels. Danazol and stanozolol[36,37], for instance, have been reported to result in an increase in plasma protein C levels, while treatment with L-asparginase[38] or oral anticoagulants[39] will result in a decrease of plasma protein C levels.

PROTEIN C ASSAYS

Two different types of assays can be used to measure the concentration of protein C in plasma: immunological assays and functional assays (for reviews see refs 40 and 41). The immunological assays include electroimmunoassays[15,16,42], ELISAs[43,44] and radioimmunoassays[45,46]. Functional assays include a variety of methods differing in concept, specificity and complexity[40,41,47]. All these assays differ in sensitivity, precision, accuracy and costs. The selection of a protein C assay for use in the daily routine therefore depends strongly on the infrastructure of the local clinical laboratory. Within the framework of the multicentre studies organized by ECAT, the initial selection of protein C assays was based on what was available in 1984. Later, other assays were added and recommended for use in the central analysis of patient samples after careful evaluation of their performance and usefulness for application in semi-automated analysis.

In the following sections those methods will be discussed in detail that were selected for the analysis of the samples in the ECAT Angina Pectoris Study. In separate sections other alternative methods will be briefly introduced and discussed.

Protein C antigen

Initially the recommended method for measuring protein C antigen was the electroimmunoassay (Laurell or rocket assay) using a locally prepared rabbit antiserum against human protein C[15]. To date anti-protein C serum is commercially available from many different manufacturers; some manufacturers even provide ready-to-use Laurell plates for the measurement of protein C antigen (Diagnostica Stago, American Diagnostics).

Principle

A fixed amount of sample is allowed to migrate in an electric field in an agarose gel containing specific anti-protein C antibodies at alkaline pH (8.8). Negatively charged proteins such as protein C will migrate towards the anode. The protein C will interact with the specific rabbit anti-protein C antibodies. These interactions will result in the formation of insoluble immunoprecipitates (precipitation peaks or rockets) after equilibrium has been established. The length of the precipitation rocket is directly related to the concentration of protein C in the plasma. The protein C antigen concentration in a test sample is determined by measuring the length of the precipitation rocket and reading the antigen content from a calibration curve which relates length of the rocket to the protein C antigen content.

Materials

The same buffer is used as gel buffer, dilution buffer and electrophoresis buffer. For 10 litres of buffer

  28.9 g Tris(hydroxymethyl)aminomethane (MW 121.10; TRIZMA Base, Sigma),
  48.8 g sodium barbital ($C_8H_{12}N_2NaO_3$) (MW 206.18; Merck),
  12.35 g barbital ($C_8H_{12}N_2O_3$) (MW 184.2; Merck),
  3.72 g EDTA ($C_{10}H_{14}N_2 \cdot 2H_2O$) (MW 372.2; Boehringer)

are added to 2 litres of distilled water; the pH is adjusted to 8.8 with 5 N NaOH; then distilled water is added to a final volume of 10 litres. The buffer should be stored at 4 °C.

Because in some clinical laboratories the use of barbital buffers is avoided, we like to recommend the following buffer as a suitable alternative:

  31.6 mmol/L Tricine (Sigma), 91.5 mmol/L Tris, 1 mmol/L EDTA (pH 8.6).

Agarose solution (1%). It is recommended that Agarose IndubioseA-37 (Pharma-Industrie IBF, Villeneuve, France) should be used. Alternative sources of agarose could be Seakem LE Agarose (FMC Bioproducts) or Agarose T (Behringwerke).

For each plate (10 × 10 cm) 120 mg of agarose is mixed with 12 ml electrophoresis buffer in a 20 ml glass tube, placed in a boiling water bath or thermo-bloc (100 °C) until complete solution of the agarose, and transferred to a thermo-bloc at 54 °C, where it is stored for at least 30 min before pouring the plates.

Preparation of the plates, electrophoresis

A glass plate (10 × 10 × 0.15 cm) or a piece of 0.2 mm Gelbond® film (FMC Bioproducts) of similar size is placed on a horizontal table. To 12 ml of 1% agarose solution (54 °C) the required amount of antiserum is added and mixed thoroughly, after which the agarose solution is poured evenly over the plate. After 10 min the solidified gel is placed in a refrigerator (4 °C) in a moist atmosphere. It should harden for at least 1 h before wells can be punched (usually 19 wells of 2 mm or 10 wells of 4 mm diameter, at about 3 cm from the edge).

Duplicate samples (4 μl in 2 mm wells or 13 μl in 4 mm wells) can be applied in balanced order. Electrophoresis time is 20 h at 120 V (7 mA/plate; on the plate 3.75 V/cm).

Staining of the plates

After electrophoresis the gels are rinsed in 0.9% NaCl for about 4 h (room temperature), pressed, dried and stained with a solution of Coomassie Brilliant Blue R250 (Serva; 2.5 g in 1 litre methanol/acetic acid/water, 5/1/5). Afterwards the excess of staining solution is removed with methanol/acetic acid/water (5/1/5). This solution is renewed repeatedly until the plate is clean. The plate is rinsed with distilled water and dried.

Calculations

The assay is calibrated with dilutions of a pooled normal plasma (1//1, 1/2, 1/4, 1/8) in electrophoresis buffer. Usually the potency of this standard is arbitrarily set to 100% or 1 unit/ml (1 unit being the amount of protein C present in 1 ml of pooled normal plasma). Some of the commercial standards have been calibrated against the first International Standard for protein C in plasma which contains 0.82 i.u. per ampoule[48].

The length of the rockets obtained for the dilutions of the standard is plotted against the concentration of protein C antigen (%, U/ml, i.u./ml) on log–log paper for the construction of the calibration curve (usually a straight line). The lengths of the rockets for test samples are read on this calibration curve by intrapolation.

Normal ranges

Among healthy volunteers protein C antigen varies between 0.65 and 1.45 units/ml (n = 33; ref. 15). In patients on oral anticoagulant treatment protein C antigen is a function of the intensity of treatment (see Table 11.1) (ref. 15).

Table 11.1 Protein C antigen during stable oral anticoagulant treatment

INR*	Protein C antigen mean	(U/ml) range
2.4–2.8	0.47 ± 0.09	0.30–0.64
2.8–3.2	0.41 ± 0.08	0.30–0.68
3.2–3.6	0.40 ± 0.08	0.30–0.68
3.6–4.0	0.43 ± 0.09	0.25–0.64
4.0–4.4	0.38 ± 0.08	0.21–0.56
>4.4	0.33 ± 0.07	0.21–0.45

* INR = International Normalized Ratio

General comments

For the electroimmunoassay of protein C antigen it is essential that EDTA is present in the gel and electrophoresis buffer. Only under these conditions will the fully carboxylated and non-carboxylated forms of protein C migrate at an identical rate. This is important because otherwise the higher mobility of the non-carboxylated protein (as present in plasmas of patients treated with oral anticoagulants) will result in relatively over-long precipitation peaks, and therefore in apparently higher protein C antigen concentrations (see refs 42 and 49). A disadvantage of the use of EDTA is that in most cases twice as much antiserum is needed to obtain the same peak height for undiluted pooled normal plasma. Good-quality rabbit anti-protein C serum can be used at concentrations between 0.5% and 2%.

The staining and destaining solutions contain methanol. If the use of methanol needs to be avoided, methanol can be replaced by ethanol (some loss in destaining efficiency).

Alternative protein C antigen assays

Many different protein C antigen assays have been described in the literature[40–46]. From these only the ELISA systems are commercially available: ELISA based on the use of rabbit anti-protein C immunoglobulins (Diagnostica Stago), ELISA based on the use of two different murine monoclonal antibodies (Organon Teknika) or isolated (conjugated) anti-protein C immunoglobulins (Dako A/S, Glostrup, Denmark). One should realize that slight differences in specificity may exist between the various protein C antigen assays, especially in clinical samples: in patients on oral anticoagulants lower protein C antigen concentrations are usually found by ELISA than by Laurell assay[49,50].

Similarly complexes between activated protein C and its plasma inhibitors are completely recovered in the Laurell assay, only for 50% in the 'polyclonal' ELISAs[49] and not at all in the monoclonal ELISA from Organon Teknika (because one of the monoclonals is directed against the active site of APC).

Protein C activity assay

The ideal protein C activity assay would be a test which measures all functional aspects of the protein C molecule (Ca^{2+} binding, activation by thrombin–thrombomodulin, interaction with protein S, proteolytic inactivation of factors Va and VIIIa). Such an assay is presently not available. On the other hand many functional protein C assays have been described in the literature[40,41,47]. In all these assays essentially three steps can be recognized.

1. Partial purification of protein C from the test sample[51-55]; this is included in most of the first-generation assays, but omitted in many of the second-generation assays.
2. Activation of protein C by thrombin alone (in the absence of Ca^{2+})[51,54], by the thrombin–thrombomodulin complex (in the presence of Ca^{2+})[52,53,55] or by the protein C activator from the venom of *Agkistrodon contortrix contortrix*[56-58].
3. Measurement of the activity of the APC formed with a spectrophotometric method (kinetic or endpoint methods) or with a clotting method[51-55].

For the first ECAT studies we selected one of the first-generation protein C activity assays. This assay was developed in our own laboratory[54] and is commercially available in a slightly modified form (Coa-set, KabiVitrum). Because this assay is rather complicated in design, laborious to perform and less suitable for semi-automated analysis, one of the second-generation tests was selected for subsequent ECAT studies (Coa-test, KabiVitrum).

Principle of the protein C activity assay (Leiden protocol)[54]

In a first step citrated plasma (supplemented with an excess protamine chloride to neutralize heparin, if present) is adsorbed with a critical concentration of $Al(OH)_3$. In this step the (fully) carboxylated protein C is adsorbed to (and later eluted from) the $Al(OH)_3$ gel and thus separated from fibrinogen, APC inhibitors, thrombin inhibitors and non-carboxylated protein C. During the second step a suitable dilution of the $Al(OH)_3$ eluate is treated with a relatively high concentration of thrombin in the absence of Ca^{2+}. After 45 min of activation protein C activation is stopped by adding an excess of heparin/antithrombin III (complete neutralization of thrombin). In the third step a sample of the activation mixture is diluted in a solution containing a chromogenic substrate reactive with APC.

The assay is calibrated with dilutions of pooled normal plasma in protein C-deficient plasma. Samples are tested either undiluted or prediluted in protein C-deficient plasma.

Materials

(a) Buffers
1. Washing buffer: 0.3 mol/L EDTA, 3 mmol/L benzamidine.

2. Elution buffer: 0.25 mol/L sodium–potassium phosphate, pH 8.0 (19 volumes of 0.25 mol/L Na_2HPO_4 plus 1 volume 0.25 mol/L KH_2PO_4).
3. Activation buffer: 0.1 mol/L Tris-HCl (pH 8.0), 0.1% bovine serum albumin (Sigma).
4. S-2366-mixture: 1 volume 50 mmol/L Tris-HCl, 0.3 mol/L NaCl (pH 8.5), 0.6 volumes H_2O, 0.2 volumes 0.1% ovalbumin (Sigma), 0.2 volumes 4 mmol/L S-2366 (KabiVitrum).

(b) Reagents

1. $Al(OH)_3$ suspension: stock suspension: 30 g $Al(OH)_3$ (BDH 27077 moist gel) in 100 ml buffer (25 mmol/L trisodium citrate $2H_2O$, 0.9% NaCl, 10 mmol/L benzamidine, pH 8.0); store at 4 °C. The working suspension is a 1:5 dilution of the stock suspension in the aforementioned buffer.
2. Thrombin buffer: 9 ml activation buffer plus 45 µl human thrombin (~ 40 µmol/L). This solution is freshly prepared before step 2 of the assay (see Test procedure, below).
3. Antithrombin III–heparin mix: 9 volumes of (semi)purified antithrombin III (~ 1.8 U/ml; free of APC inhibitors!) plus 0.1 volume of heparin (Thromboliquine, Organon BV, Oss; 5000 i.u./ml).
4. Protein C-deficient plasma: this plasma can be prepared by affinity chromatography of normal plasma over anti-protein C IgG-Sepharose (54). It is also commercially available as a lyophilized plasma (Diagnostica Stago, Behringwerke).

Test procedure

(a) Preparation of eluates. One millilitre plasma – supplemented with 10 µl protamine chloride (10 mg/ml) – is mixed with 200 µl $Al(OH)_3$ suspension in conic 1.2 ml Eppendorf tubes for 30 min at room temperature using a shaker or rotator. The suspension is then centrifuged at room temperature (Microfuge; 5 min; 12 000 rpm). The supernatant is removed carefully and can be discarded. The precipitate is suspended in 800 µl washing buffer and centrifuged (see above). The supernatant is removed and the precipitate resuspended in 200 µl elution buffer, incubated for 20 min in a shaker (at room temperature) and centrifuged (see above). The supernatant (eluate) is transferred to a fresh tube; eluates can be used directly or stored at −20 °C.

(b) Activation of eluates. Thirty microlitres of eluate is added to 200 µl of thrombin buffer and incubated in a plastic tube for 45 min at 37 °C. Then 30 µl of the antithrombin III–heparin mix is added and incubated for a further 15 min at 37 °C.

(c) Assay of activated protein C. Fifty microlitres of the activation mix is added to 600 µl of the prewarmed S-2366 mix (in a plastic tube) and incubated for 45 min at 37 °C. After the further addition of 300 µl of 50% acetic acid the absorbance is read at 405 nm.

Calibration curve

The calibration curve (100%, 75%, 50%, 30%, 10%, 0%) is made by diluting pooled normal plasma (100% or 1 unit/ml) in protein C-deficient plasma. This curve should be included in each assay. In each assay a control plasma is also included. We used a pool of plasmas of patients on oral anticoagulant treatment (check on separation of carboxylated and non-carboxylated protein C during the first step). The protein C concentration of test samples should always be read on the calibration curve that was included in that particular test series (steps (a)–(c)).

Normal ranges

In healthy volunteers protein C activity ranges from 0.61 to 1.32 U/ml, while the protein C activity/antigen ratios vary from 0.64 to 1.57[54].

In patients on oral anticoagulant treatment protein C activity varies with the intensity of the treatment[54].

Alternative methods

As mentioned previously, the discovery of a specific protein C activator (Protac®) in the venom of *Agkistrodon contortrix contortrix*[59–61] resulted in a second generation of protein C activity assays. Because the activity of Protac® is not dependent on Ca^{2+} ions, and is insensitive to plasma protease inhibitors, Protac® can be used to activate protein C directly in plasma; during a second incubation the activity of the APC formed can be quantitated with a spectrophotometric or clotting technique. For the ECAT studies we replaced the three-step adsorption step (Leiden assay) that was used in the first study by a two-step snake venom test (kinetic mode of CoaTest, KabiVitrum). Figure 11.1 shows that there is excellent agreement between these two methods in plasmas of individuals not using oral anticoagulants. Several manufacturers distribute very similar protein C activity tests. All these tests use different chromogenic substrates for the measurement of APC. Some of these tests have been used and evaluated in comparative studies[48,49,58,62,63]. Most of these tests have both endpoint and kinetic modifications. For several reasons the author prefers kinetic versions of the test. One of these reasons is that it is sometimes impossible to have a satisfactory blank in the endpoint method (see for further discussion ref. 47).

Protein C activity in patients on oral anticoagulant treatment

From international collaborative studies it has become clear that the different types of protein C activity assays can all be used for the measurement of functional protein C in the plasma of patients not treated with oral anticoagulants[48,64]. However, in plasma of a patient on oral anticoagulant treatment the actual protein C activity concentration will depend largely on the method used[40,47,49]. The main reason for this is that the protein C activators used – Protac® or thrombin–(thrombomodulin) – cleave both the

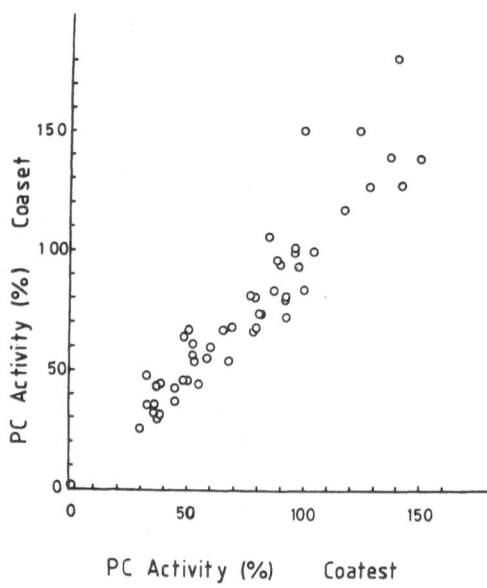

Figure 11.1 Protein C activity (CoaSet and CoaTest) in healthy individuals

carboxylated and non-carboxylated forms of protein C. The effect on the test result will then largely depend on the design of the test (cf. Figure 11.2). In the Leiden assay (three-step adsorption assay) non-carboxylated protein C is separated from the carboxylated protein C during the first step (Al(OH)$_3$ – adsorption). In this type of assay the concentration of carboxylated protein C is measured. This parameter will vary largely with the intensity of the treatment (much more so than the protein C antigen concentration) and also the ratio carboxylated protein C/total protein C will decrease with increasing intensity of treatment. In the so-called snake venom assays both the carboxylated and the non-carboxylated forms of protein C are activated by Protac®. In the spectrophotometric snake venom assay one would therefore expect that the protein C activity concentration would be equal to the protein C antigen concentration. For most assays, however, the actual measured protein C activity levels lie somewhere between the protein C activity as measured with the Leiden assay (carboxylated protein C) and the protein C antigen assay (total protein C), indicating that possibly the activation of non-carboxylated protein C (ncPC) is not complete, or that the yield of ncAPC in the assay is different from that of APC. In the anticoagulant snake venom assay the amount of APC formed is quantitated by measuring its effect on a global clotting time like the APTT which is sensitive to factor V and factor VIII. With this type of assay the measured protein C activity levels are much lower than that found with the Leiden assay. This may be explained by assuming that ncAPC will behave as a competitive inhibitor of APC in the APTT test (for instance by still binding to protein S). Altogether, one has to be very careful in selecting a protein C activity assay for application in a routine clinical laboratory, especially when many samples of patients

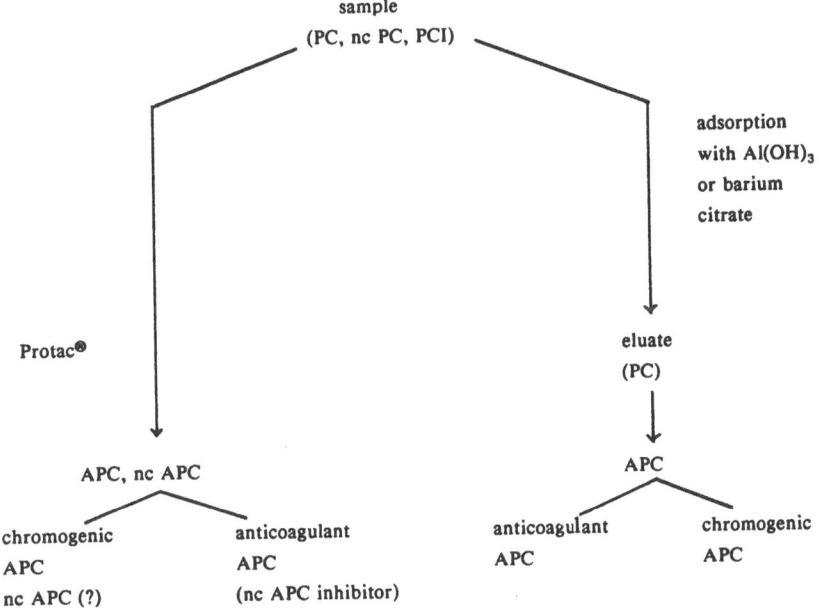

Figure 11.2 Design of protein C activity assays. (nc) PC (non-carboxylated) PC; nc APC (non-carboxylated) APC; PCI, protein C inhibitors

on oral anticoagulants are offered for analysis. The use of functional protein C assays for the laboratory diagnosis of hereditary protein C deficiency therefore still needs further evaluation[22].

References

1. Esmon CT. Protein C: biochemistry, physiology and clinical implications. Blood 1983; 62: 1155–8.
2. Stenflo J. The biochemistry of protein C. In: Bertina RM, ed. Protein C and related proteins. Edinburgh: Churchill Livinstone, 1988; 21–54.
3. Sills RH, Marlar RA, Montgomery RR, Desphande GN, Humbert JR. Severe homozygous protein C deficiency. J Pediat 1984; 105: 409–13.
4. Marlar RA, Kleiss AJ, Griffin JH. Mechanism of action of human activated protein C, a thrombin-dependent anticoagulant enzyme. Blood 1982; 59: 1067–72.
5. Walker FJ. Protein S and the regulation of activated protein C. Sem Thromb Hemostas 1984; 10: 131–8.
6. Koedam JA, Meijers JCM, Sixma JJ, Bouma BN. Inactivation of human factor VIII by activated protein C. J Clin Invest 1988; 82: 1236–43.
7. Suzuki K, Stenflo J, Dahlbäck B, Teodorsson B. Inhibition of human coagulation factor V by activated protein C. J Biol Chem 1983; 258: 1914–20.
8. Esmon CT. The roles of protein C and thrombomodulin in the regulation of blood coagulation. J Biol Chem 1989; 264: 4743–6.
9. Esmon NL, De Bault LE, Esmon CT. Proteolytic formation and properties of γ-carboxyglutamic acid – domainless protein C. J Biol Chem 1983; 258: 5548–53.
10. Suzuki N, Nishioka J, Hashimoto S. Protein C inhibitor. Purification from human plasma and characterization. J Biol Chem 1983; 258: 163–8.

11. Van der Meer FJM, van Tilburg NH, van Wijngaarden A, van der Linden IK, Briët E, Bertina RM. A second plasma inhibitor of activated protein C: α_1-antitrypsin. Thromb Haemostas 1989; 62: 756–62.
12. Heeb MJ, Gruber A, Griffin JH. Metal ion dependent inhibition of activated protein C by α_2 macroglobulin and α_2-antiplasmin in human blood. Arteriosclerosis 1990; 10: 893a.
13. Marlar RA, Montgomery RR, Broekmans AW. Diagnosis and treatment of homozygous protein C deficiency. J Pediat 1989; 114: 528–34.
14. Marlar RA, Neumann A. Neonatal purpura fulminans due to homozygous protein C or protein S deficiencies. Sem. Thromb. 1990; 16: 299–309.
15. Bertina RM, Broekmans AW, van der Linden IK, Mertens K. Protein C deficiency in a Dutch family with thrombotic disease. Thromb Haemostas 1982; 48: 1–5.
16. Griffin JH, Evatt B, Zimmerman TS, Kleiss AJ, Wideman C. Deficiency of protein C in congenital thrombotic disease. J Clin Invest 1981; 68: 1370–3.
17. Broekmans AW, Conard J. Hereditary protein C deficiency. In: Bertina RM, ed. Protein C and related proteins. Edinburgh: Churchill Livingstone, 1988; 160–81.
18. Gladson CL, Scharrer I, Hack V, Beck KH, Griffin JH. The frequency of type I heterozygous protein S and protein C deficiency in 141 unrelated young patients with venous thrombosis. Thromb Haemostas 1988; 59: 18–22.
19. Bertina RM. Prevalence of hereditary thrombophilia and the identification of genetic risk factors. Fibrinolysis 1988; 2(S2): 7–13.
20. Seligsohn U, Berger A, Abend M, Rubin I, Attias D, Zivelin A, Rapaport SI. Homozygous protein C deficiency manifested by massive venous thrombosis in the newborn. N Engl J Med 1984; 310: 559–62.
21. Miletich J, Sherman L, Broze G Jr. Absence of thrombosis in subjects with heterozygous protein C deficiency. N Engl J Med 1987; 317: 991–6.
22. Pabinger I, Kyrle PA, Speiser W, Stoffels U, Jung M, Lechner K. Diagnosis of protein C deficiency in patients on oral anticoagulant treatment: comparison of three different functional protein C assays. Thromb Haemostas 1990; 63: 407–12.
23. Pabinger I. Lechner K. Acquired protein C and protein S deficiency. In: Bertina RM, ed. Protein C and related proteins. Edinburgh: Churchill Livingstone, 1988; 213–25.
24. Cohen H, Mackie U, Walshe K, Gillmer MD, Machin SJ. A comparison of the effects of two triphasic oral contraceptives on haemostasis. Br J Haemotol 1988; 69: 259–63.
25. Gensini GF, Rostagno C, Abbat R, Favilla S, Mannucci PM, Serneri GGN, Bonomi AB. Increased protein C and fibrinopeptide A concentration in patients with angina. Thromb Res 1988; 30: 517–25.
26. Cosio FG, Harker C, Batard MA, Brandt JT, Griffin JH. Plasma concentrations of the natural anticoagulants protein C and protein S in patients with proteinuria. J Lab Clin Med 1985; 106: 218–22.
27. Pabinger-Fasching I, Lechner K, Niessner H, Schmidt P, Balzar E, Mannhalter CL. High levels of plasma protein C in nepthrotic syndrome. Thromb Haemostas 1985; 53: 5–7.
28. Blamey SL, Lowe GDO, Bertina RM, Kluft C, Sue Ling HM, Davies JA, Fobes CD. Protein C antigen levels in major abdominal surgery: relationships of deep vein thrombosis, malignancy and treatment with stanozolol. Thromb Haemostas 1985; 54: 622–5.
29. Vigano S, Mannucci PM, D'Aangelo A, Gelfi C, Gensini GF, Rostagno C, Serneri GGN. The significance of protein C antigen in acute and chronic liver biliary disease. Am J Clin Pathol 1984; 84: 454–8.
30. Marlar RA, Endres-Brooks J, Miller C. Serial studies of protein C and its plasma inhibitor in patients with disseminated intravascular coagulation. Blood 1985; 66: 59–63.
31. Ceriello A, Quatrano A, Dello Russo P, Marchi E, Barbanti M, Rita Milani M, Giugliano D. Protein C deficiency in insulin-dependent diabetes: a hyperglycemia-related phenomenon. Thromb Haemostas 1990; 64: 104–7.
32. Vukovich TC, Schernthaner G. Decreased protein C levels in patients with insulin-dependent type I diabetes mellitus. Diabetes 1986; 35: 617–19.
33. Kloczko J, Wojtukiewicz M, Bielawiec M, Borowska M. Reduced protein C levels in patients with essential hypertension. Thromb Haemostas 1987; 58: 793.
34. Green D, Scott JP. Is sickle cell crisis a thrombotic event. Am J Hematol 1986; 23: 317–21.
35. Miletich JP. Laboratory diagnosis of protein C deficiency. Sem Thromb Haemostas 1990; 16: 169–76.

36. Gonzalez R, Alberca I, Sala N, Vicente V. Protein C deficiency – response to danazol and DDAVP. Thromb Haemostas 1985; 53: 320–2.
37. Broekmans AW, Conard J, van Weijenberg RG, Horellou MH, Kluft C, Bertina RM. Treatment of hereditary protein C deficiency with stanozolol. Thromb Haemostas 1987; 57: 20–4.
38. Conard J, Horellou MH, Dreden P, Potevin F, Zittoun R, Samama M. Decrease in protein C in L-asparaginase-treated patients. Br J Haematol 1985; 59: 725–41.
39. Vigano S, Mannucci PM, Solinas S, Botasso B, Mariani G. Decrease in protein C antigen and formation of an abnormal protein soon after starting oral anticoagulant therapy. Br J Haematol 1984; 57: 213–20.
40. Bertina RM. Assays for protein C. In: Bertina RM, ed. Protein C and related proteins. Edinburgh: Churchill Livingstone, 1988; 130–50.
41. Marlar RA, Adcock DM. Clinical evaluation of protein C: a comparative review of antigenic and functional assays. Progr Pathol 1989; 20: 1040–7.
42. Mikami S, Tuddenham EGD. Studies on immunological assay of vitamin K-dependent factors II. Comparison of four immunoassay methods with functional activity of protein C in human plasma. Br J Haematol 1986; 62: 183–93.
43. Boyer C, Rothschild C, Wolf M, Amiral J, Meyer D, Larrieu MJ. A new method for the estimation of protein C by ELISA. Thromb Res 1984; 36: 579–89.
44. Suzuki K, Moriguchi A, Nagayoshi A, Mutoh S, Katszuki S, Hashimoto S. Enzyme immunoassay of human protein C by using monoclonal antibodies. Thromb Res 1985; 38: 611–21.
45. Ikeda K, Stenflo J. A radioimmunoassay for protein C. Thromb Res 1985; 39: 297–306.
46. Epstein DJ, Bergum PW, Bajaj SP, Rapaport SI. Radioimmunoassay for protein C and factor X. Plasma antigen levels in abnormal haemostatic states. Am J Clin Pathol 1984; 82: 573–81.
47. Bertina RM. Specificity of protein C and protein S assays. Res Clin Lab 1990; 20: 127–38.
48. Hubbard AR. Standardization of protein C in plasma: establishment of an International Standard. Thromb Haemostas 1988; 59: 464–7.
49. Bertina RM. An International Collaborative study on the performance of protein C antigen assays. Thromb Haemostas 1987; 57: 112–17.
50. Mannucci PM, Boyer C, Tripodi A, Vigano d'Angelo S, Wolf M, Valsecchi C, d'Angelo A, Meyer D and Larrieu MJ. Multicenter comparison of five functional and two immunological assays for protein C. Thromb Haemostas 1987; 57: 44–8.
51. Francis RB, Patch MJ. A functional assay for protein C in human plasma. Thromb Res 1983; 32: 605–13.
52. Comp PC, Nixon RR, Esmon CT. Determination of functional levels of protein C, an antithrombotic protein, using thrombin–thrombomodulin complex. Blood 1984; 63: 15–21.
53. Sala N, Owen NG, Collen D. Functional assay of protein C in human plasma. Blood 1984; 63: 671–5.
54. Bertina RM, Broekmans AW, Krommenhoek-van Es C, van Wijngaarden A. The use of a functional and immunologic assay for plasma protein C in the study of the heterogeneity of congenital protein C deficiency. Thromb Haemostas 1984; 51: 1–5.
55. Vigano-D'Angelo S, Comp PC, Esmon CT, D'Angelo A. Relationship between protein C antigen and anticoagulant activity during oral anti-coagulation and in selected disease states, J Clin Invest 1986; 77: 416–25.
56. Martinoli JL, Stocker K. Fast functional protein C assay using Protac, a novel protein C activator. Thromb Res 1986; 43: 253–64.
57. Francis RB, Seyfert U. Rapid amidolytic assay of protein C in whole plasma using an activator from the venom of Agkistrodon contortrix contortrix. Am J Clin Pathol 1987; 87: 619–25.
58. Vinazzer H, Pangraz U. Protein C: comparison of different assays in normal and abnormal plasma samples. Thromb Res 1987; 46: 1–8.
59. Stocker K, Fischer H, Meier J, Brogli M, Svendsen L. Protein C activators in snake venoms. Behring Institut Mitteilungen 1986; 79: 37–47.
60. Exner T, Vaasjoki R. Characterization and some properties of the protein C activator from Agkistrodon contortrix contortrix venom. Thromb Haemostas 1988; 59: 40–4.
61. Orthner CL, Bhattacharya P, Strickland DK. Characterization of a protein C activator from the venom of *Agkistrodon contortrix contortrix*. Biochemistry 1988; 27: 2558–64.

62. Sturk A, Morrien-Salomons WM, Huisman MV, Borm JJJ, Büller HR, ten Cate JW. Analytical and clinical evaluation of commercial protein C assays. Clin Chim Acta 1987; 165: 263–70.
63. Franchi F, Tripodi A, Valsecchi C, Mannucci PM. Functional assays of protein C: comparison of two snake-venom assays with two thrombin assays. Thromb Haemostas 1988; 60: 145–7.
64. Mannucci PM, Boyer C, Tripodi A, Vigano-D'Angelo S, Wolf M, Valsecchi C, D'Angelo A, Meyer D, Larrieu MJ. Multicenter Comparison of five functional and two immunologic assays for protein C. Thromb Haemostas 1987; 57: 44–8.

12
Protein S antigen

R. M. BERTINA

INTRODUCTION

Protein S is a vitamin K-dependent plasma glycoprotein (MW 70 000)[1,2]. Unlike the other vitamin K-dependent coagulation factors protein S is not the zymogen of a serine protease. Apart from a domain rich in γ-carboxyglutamic acid residues (Gla-domain), a thrombin-sensitive region (TSR), and four epidermal-growth-factor like domains (EGF domains), protein S contains a large carboxyterminal domain homologous to the rat androgen-binding protein (ABP) and the human sex hormone-binding globulin (SHBG)[3]. Protein S is synthesized in the liver, endothelial cells and megakaryocytes[4-6]. The biological half-life of protein S[7] is about 42.5 h. In pooled normal plasma the total protein S concentration is about 25 µg/ml (0.36 µmol/L).

Physiological role

Protein S is the protein cofactor of the anticoagulant enzyme activated protein C (APC) and therefore is an essential component of the protein C anticoagulant pathway[8]. It stimulates the inactivation of factor Va and factor VIIIa by APC both in plasma and purified systems[9-12]. It is also required for the expression of the profibrinolytic effect of APC in a whole blood clot lysis system[13]. Protein S forms a 1:1 complex with APC on phospholipid surfaces and is thus thought to stimulate the phospholipid-dependent inactivation of factors Va and VIIIa.

The APC cofactor activity of protein S is regulated by two independent processes. First, protein S is cleaved by thrombin in the TSR region; this cleavage results in the formation of a molecule consisting of two chains linked by one disulphide bridge, which no longer has APC cofactor activity[14,15]. However, under physiological conditions (i.e. in the presence of Ca^{2+}) this reaction is rather slow, and therefore will require high local thrombin concentrations.

99

A second mechanism controlling the APC cofactor activity of protein S is its ability to form a 1:1 complex with the C4b binding protein (C4bBP), an important regulatory component of the complement system[16-18]. The C4bBP protein S complex has no APC cofactor activity[19,20]. However, this complex – which can still bind to phospholipid membranes – may play a role in the regulation of complement activation[21].

In citrated human plasma or in serum, free and C4bBP–protein S occur in a ratio of 2:3[16,20,22]. This distribution would fit with the distribution calculated on basis of the K_d reported for the C4bBP–protein S complex (0.9×10^{-7}, see ref. 17). However, recent binding studies[18] report a 100-fold lower K_d for the complex in the presence of Ca^{2+}. Extrapolation of these data to the physiological situation suggests that all protein S would be in the complexed form. The fact that this clearly is not the case prompted Dahlbäck et al. to postulate the existence of a novel regulatory element in the C4bBP–protein S interaction[18,21]. The binding of protein S to C4bBP occurs via a separate unique subunit of C4bBP (β subunit)[23].

Pathophysiological aspects

Hereditary defects

The importance of protein S for the control of thrombin formation in vivo is most dramatically demonstrated in neonates who are homozygotes or double heterozygotes for hereditary protein S deficiency[24]. Such patients develop, shortly after birth, clinical symptoms (among others purpura fulminans syndrome) that are very similar to those reported for homozygous protein C deficiency[25]. Heterozygotes for hereditary protein S deficiency have an increased risk for the development of venous thrombosis at relatively young age[26-28]. Recently several reports have been published suggesting that protein S deficiency may also predispose to juvenile arterial thrombosis[29,30]. However, this possible relationship will need further evaluation.

In plasma protein S circulates both as free and C4bBP-complexed protein S. This will complicate the laboratory diagnosis of hereditary protein S deficiencies. In fact three types of deficiencies have been recognized[31]. In type I protein S deficiency there is a reduction of total protein S antigen till about 50% of normal[22,27]. Type I deficiencies are caused by alterations in the protein S gene that do not permit normal transcription, translation and/or secretion of the protein[32]. In type II protein S deficiency the total protein S antigen is normal, while one of the protein S genes makes a molecule with a strongly reduced biological activity. In the laboratory this deficiency can be diagnosed by the reduced ratio protein S activity/free protein S antigen[31,33]. So far only one family with a hereditary type II protein S deficiency has been reported[33]. The third type of hereditary protein S deficiency is the so-called type III deficiency[31]. In patients with this type of deficiency the free protein S antigen is lower than expected on the basis of the concentrations of total protein S and C4bBP. The molecular basis of this defect is still unsolved (defect in protein S or in C4bBP?). It should be noted that in the nomenclature originally proposed by Comp et al.[34] a type I deficiency is identical to our type III deficiency, while their type II deficiency is identical to our type I deficiency.

Acquired abnormalities

Abnormal plasma levels of total and/or free protein S have been reported for a number of clinical conditions. Sometimes the interpretation of the reported data is hampered by the lack of information on the specificity of the assay (especially true for some of the total PS antigen assays).

Reduced levels of total protein S have been reported for patients using oral anticoagulants[7,27], during pregnancy and use of oral contraceptives[36-38] and in patients with liver disease[22]. Conflicting data (reduced/increased PS antigen) have been reported for patients with diabetes mellitus[35,39]. Increased PS antigen (total) has been found in patients with nephrotic syndrome[40]. The simultaneous increase in C4bBP, however, might result in an acquired deficiency of free protein S[41]. No change in total protein S antigen has been observed during DIC[7,22].

Under conditions in which acute phase reactions may occur, elevated C4bBP levels might cause a reduction in free protein S concentration. This may occur during an acute thrombotic episode, although elevated total and free protein S antigen also have been reported for acute deep-vein thrombosis[42].

PROTEIN S ASSAYS

The development of suitable assays for the measurement of protein S in plasma is severely hampered by the fact that protein S circulates in the plasma both as free protein S and as the C4bBP–protein S complex[16]. The distribution of protein S over the free and complexed form is dictated by the total concentrations of protein S and C4bBP, the apparent equilibrium constant and the concentration of other – still unknown – ligands for one of the components of the reaction, that will influence the apparent K_d of the C4bBP–protein S complexes[17,18].

Basically three types of assays can be recognized:

1. immunological assays for total protein S,
2. immunological assays for free protein S,
3. protein S functional assays.

For the ECAT studies it was decided to include the measurement of total protein S antigen, because at that time the development of functional protein S assays had just started in highly specialized research institutes. To date several protein S activity assays have been reported[7,20,43-46] and some of these are even available commercially. So far the performance of these assays has not been evaluated in international collaborative studies.

Several immunological assays for the measurement of total protein S in plasma have been reported: Laurell types of assay[20,27], immunoradiometric assays[22,47], ELISAs[48-51] and RIAs[52,53]. The selection of a suitable assay was made on the basis of sensitivity and specificity. The demonstration that free and complexed protein S are measured with the same efficiency (i.e. protein S concentration is independent of the actual C4bBP concentration) is an especially important criterion for selection of a total protein S antigen assay. In some of the Laurell assays two different precipitation peaks are observed for free and complexed protein S, which makes it impossible to read the total protein S concentration[43,54]. Also, when EIA, ELISA or RIA systems are used, it is important to check whether the further addition of C4bBP to a protein S containing sample will effect the response in the assay system[37,22,53].

The assay for total protein S antigen that was selected for the ECAT studies is an ELISA for total protein S antigen[48] which may be considered as a modification of the immunoradiometric assays previously reported from our laboratory[22,47].

Principle of the ELISA for total protein S

Wells of microtitre plates are coated with rabbit antibodies against human protein S. During the first incubation these immobilized antibodies (catching antibodies) will react with the protein S molecules present in the sample (dilutions). After the establishment of an equilibrium the wells are emptied, washed and incubated with a suitable dilution of anti-protein S antibodies conjugated to horseradish peroxidase (HRP) (tagging antibody). The amount of conjugate bound to the wells will be directly related to the amount of immobilized protein S and thus to the concentration of protein S in the sample (dilution). The amount of immobilized conjugate is measured during a third incubation, where the amount of immobilized HRP is measured from its reactivity towards a specific substrate (expressed in Δ absorbance/min). In this way it is possible to plot the Δ absorbance/min versus total protein S concentration (dilutions of pooled normal plasma) and to use this calibration curve to read the concentration of total protein S for the test samples by intrapolation.

Materials

ELISA buffer

This buffer is used for making the dilutions of the samples, for washing the microtitre plates, and as diluent for the anti-protein S conjugate. It consists of: 0.67 mmol/L $Na_2HPO_4 . 2H_2O$, 14 mmol/L KH_2PO_4, 0.1% (v/v) Tween 20 (pH 7.5). This solution is freshly prepared for each series of tests.

Coating buffer

This buffer is used for the coating of microtitre plates. It consists of 0.1 mol/L $NaHCO_3$, 0.5 mol/L NaCl (pH 9.0).

Substrate buffer

This buffer is used to dissolve the HRP substrate OPD (ortho-phenylene-diamine). It consists of 22.2 mmol/L citric acid, 51.4 mmol/L $NaH_2PO_4 \cdot H_2O$ (pH 5.0) and can be stored for several weeks at 4 °C.

Substrate solution

Ortho-phenylene-diamine (dihydrochloride) (Sigma 20 mg) is dissolved in 50 ml substrate buffer (see above). About 1 min before addition to the microtitre plates 20 µl of a 30% H_2O_2 solution is added. This volume of substrate solution should be sufficient for four or five plates.

Stop-reagent

4 N H_2SO_4 is used to stop the peroxidase-catalysed conversion of OPD.

Catching antibody

As catching antibody rabbit antibodies against human protein S are used; routinely these antibodies are obtained by isolating the non-Ca(II) dependent fraction of the anti-protein S antibodies from the antiserum by immunoaffinity chromatography on protein S Sepharose (2 mg purified human protein S/ml gel)[22,47]. Stock solutions (>0.050 mg IgG/ml) are stored in 1 ml aliquots at −20 °C.

Tagging antibody

The same non-Ca(II)-dependent anti-protein S antibodies that are used as catching antibodies are used as tagging antibodies. Horseradish peroxidase (HRP) is coupled to the anti-protein S IgG using the reagent *N*-succinimidyl 3-(2-piridylthio)propionate (SPDP), as described elsewhere[55]. The conjugate is stored in suitable aliquots at −20 °C in a buffer containing 0.3 mol/L NaCl. Dilutions of the conjugate (usually ~1/4000) are prepared about 30 min prior to use. It should be noted that anti-protein S HRP conjugate can be purchased from Dako A/S (Glostrup, Denmark).

Titertek assay plates

These were purchased from Titertek (Immuno-Assay plates). Other plates may be used only after careful analysis of their suitability for this assay (homogeneity of plates, coating performance, background absorbance).

Other materials

For the transfer of samples, conjugate, or substrate solution to the microtitre plate multichannel pipettes are used. Absorbances are read on a multichannel analyser (Titertek Multiscan Plus) using a filter of 492 nm.

Test procedure

Coating of microtitre plates

This is performed by incubating the wells with 110 µl/well of the catching antibody (>4 µg/ml in coating buffer) at 4 °C. Plates are sealed with parafilm and stored at 4 °C for periods of up to 1 month. Minimal time required for coating is overnight at 4 °C.

Prior to the actual test, sufficient plates are removed from the stock. The coating solution is carefully removed, after which the plates are repeatedly washed with ELISA buffer (five times). Subsequently, wells are incubated with 150 µl of a solution of 2% bovine serum albumin (Sigma) in ELISA buffer (30 min at room temperature), and washed five times with ELISA buffer.

Test protocol

Suitable dilutions of test sample and standard (100 µl) are added to the wells and incubated for 18 h (usually overnight) at room temperature to allow for equilibrium distribution of protein S over solid and fluid phase. Assay plates then are washed five times with ELISA buffer before 100 µl/well of a dilution of HRP-labelled anti-protein S immunoglobulin is added (usually a 1/4000 dilution of the stock in ELISA buffer). Plates are then incubated for about 45 min at room temperature. Subsequently plates are emptied and washed five times with ELISA buffer. Then 100 µl/well of substrate solution (see Substrate solution, above) is added. Plates are incubated for about 30 min (till sufficient colour has been formed) before the peroxidase activity is stopped by the addition of 100 µl/well of $4 NH_2SO_4$. Finally the absorbance at 492 nm is read in a multichannel analyser (see Other materials, above).

Calibration

The ELISA for total protein S antigen is calibrated with dilutions of pooled normal plasma (usually from 1/500 serially to 1/32 000). Routinely, samples from patients not using oral anticoagulants are tested in 1/2000 and 1/4000 dilutions, while plasmas of patients using oral anticoagulants are tested in 1/1000 and 1/2000 dilutions. Each dilution is tested in duplicate. All dilutions are made in ELISA buffer. To calculate the amount of total protein S antigen in plasmas, the absorbance values were read from the standard curve which was obtained of a least-square fit of third-order polynomial to the data plotted on a double logarithmic scale. Test results are valid when the SD is less than 10%.

At present there is no international plasma standard protein S available. Therefore each laboratory relies on its own pooled plasma. Care should be taken that sufficient individual donations have been included in the pool (plasmas of females using oral contraceptives should not be included). Total protein S antigen is expressed as a percentage or in units/ml, where 1 unit reflects the amount of protein S present in 1 ml pooled normal plasma.

Normal ranges

Using the ELISA described above, total protein S antigen was measured in 40 healthy volunteers; mean protein S antigen was 1.12 ± 0.16 unit/ml, while individual values ranged from 0.77 to 1.44 unit/ml.

In 40 patients using oral anticoagulant treatment mean protein S antigen was 0.52 ± 0.10 unit/ml, while individual values ranged from 0.34 to 0.69 units/ml. For the laboratory diagnosis of hereditary protein S deficiency, often the criterion is used that total protein S antigen should be lower than the lower limit as observed in control groups of healthy volunteers or patients treated with oral anticoagulants.

Alternative methods for the measurement of protein S antigen

As mentioned previously, total protein S antigen can also be measured by immunoradiometric assay or radio-immunoassay (see ref. 20). Moreover, several other ELISA procedures have been described in the literature[48-51], occasionally without providing sufficient details on the specificity of the test (and sensitivity to C4bBP levels). In general this is also true for the one commercial ELISA test (Diagnostica Stago) and the commercially available ready-to-use Laurell plates (Diagnostica Stago; American Diagnostics). The general performance of these commercial tests is presently evaluated in an international collaborative study organized under the auspices of the SSC subcommittee on protein C and protein S.

A general problem in using a Laurell assay for the measurement of total protein S is to devise conditions (antiserum, buffer system, electrophoresis conditions) where plasma protein S will give one single precipitation peak that really reflects the concentration of total protein S (i.e. it will not decrease after addition of excess C4bBP to a test plasma (cf. ref. 37)). Presently there are no general guidelines available. From the commercial Laurell tests for protein S, the test of Diagnostica Stago seems to fulfil the above criterion.

MEASUREMENT OF FREE PROTEIN S ANTIGEN

As previously discussed, protein S and C4bBP form a complex under physiological conditions. In plasma (citrated, or EDTA) about 40% of the total protein S is free while the remaining 60% is bound to C4bBP. Because the latter complex has no APC-cofactor activity, it is of interest to know what part of the total protein S antigen is actually free. Qualitatively this information can be obtained by using two-dimensional immunoelectrophoresis: because free protein S moves faster in the electric field than the protein S–C4bBP complexes, the distribution of total protein S over the free and bound form can be estimated from the areas under the respective precipitation peaks[34]. More quantitative information can be obtained by separating free protein S from C4bBP–protein S complexes by precipitation with polyethylene glycol[53,54]. After centrifugation the free protein S is still in the supernatant, while the complexes can be recovered from the precipitate. Two different protocols are most widely used today: in the method described by Comp *et al.*[34] PEG 6000 is used at a final concentration of 3.75%, while in the Malm protocol[53] the final concentration of PEG 6000 is 5%. The measurement of free protein S antigen in a PEG supernatant sometimes creates a problem when a protein S antigen test is used that is not really specific for total protein S (e.g. non-parallel dilution curves in ELISA systems or Laurell systems). Therefore most authors express the concentration of free protein S antigen as a percentage of the free instead of the total protein S antigen present in pooled normal plasma.

However, when using an ELISA for total protein S antigen, as described above, it is possible to express the concentration of free protein S antigen directly in units/ml by reading the absorbances on the calibration curve obtained with dilutions of pooled normal plasma (completely parallel dilution curves). In this way we found in a group of 40 healthy volunteers a mean free protein S antigen of 0.42 ± 0.13 unit/ml (range 0.23–0.78 unit/ml), while in a group of 40 patients on oral anticoagulant treatment mean free protein S antigen was 0.14 ± 0.07 unit/ml (range: 0.06–0.34 units/ml).

References

1. Di Scipio RG, Hermodson MA, Yates SG, Davie EW. A comparison of human prothrombin, factor IX, factor X and protein S. Biochemistry 1977; 16: 696–706.
2. Di Scipio RG, Davie EW. Characterization of protein S, a γ-carboxyglutamic acid containing protein from bovine and human plasma. Biochemistry 1979; 18: 899–904.
3. Lundwall A, Dackowski W, Cohen E, Schaffer M, Mahr A, Dahlbäck B, Stenflo J. Isolation and sequence of the c-DNA for human protein S, a regulator of blood coagulation. Proc Natl Acad Sci USA 1987; 83: 6716–20.
4. Fair DS, Marlar RA. Biosynthesis and secretion of factor VII, protein C, protein S and the protein C inhibitor from a human hepatoma cell-line. Blood 1986; 67: 64–70.
5. Stern D, Brett J, Harris K, Nawroth P. Participation of endothelial cells in the protein C-protein S anticoagulant pathway: the synthesis and release of protein S. J Cell Biol 1986; 102: 1971–8.
6. Ogura M, Tanabe N, Nishioka J, Suzuki K, Saito H. Biosynthesis and secretion of functional protein S by a human megakaryoblastic cell line (MEG-01). Blood 1987; 70: 301–6.
7. D'Angelo A, Vigano-D'Angelo S, Esmon CT, Comp PC. Acquired deficiencies of protein S. J Clin Invest 1988; 81: 1445–54.
8. Walker FJ. The regulation of activated protein C by a new protein; a possible function for bovine protein S. J Biol Chem 1980; 255: 5521–4.
9. Walker FJ. Regulation of activated protein C by protein S. The role of phospholipid in factor Va inactivation. J Biol Chem 1981; 256: 11128–31.
10. Walker FJ, Chavin SI, Fay PJ. Inactivation of factor VIII by activated protein C and protein S. Arch Biochem Biophys 1987; 252: 322–8.
11. Koedam JA, Meyers JCM, Sixma JJ, Bouma BM. Inactivation of human factor VIII by activated protein C. Cofactor activity of protein S and protective effect of von Willebrand factor. J Clin Invest 1988; 82: 1236–43.
12. Walker FJ. Protein S and the regulation of activated protein C. Sem Thromb Haemostas 1984; 10: 131–8.
13. De Fouw NJ, Haverkate F, Bertina RM, Koopman J, van Wijngaarden A, van Hinsbergh VWM. The cofactor role of protein S in the acceleration of whole blood clot lysis by activated protein C in vitro. Blood 1986; 67: 1189–92.
14. Walker FJ. Regulation of vitamin K dependent protein S. Inactivation by thrombin. J Biol Chem 1984; 259: 10335–9.
15. Sugo T, Dahlbäck B, Holmgren A, Stenflo J. Calcium binding of bovine protein S. Effect

of thrombin cleavage and removal of the γ-carboxyglutamic acid-containing region. J Biol Chem 1986; 261: 5116–20.

16. Dahlbäck B, Stenflo J. High molecular weight complex in human plasma between vitamin K dependent protein S and complement component C4b-binding protein. Proc Natl Acad Sci USA 1981; 78: 2512–16.

17. Dahlbäck B. Purification of human C4b-binding protein and formation of its complex with vitamin K-dependent protein S. Biochem J 1983; 209: 847–56.

18. Dahlbäck B, Frohm B, Nelsestuen G. High affinity interaction between C4b-binding protein and vitamin K-dependent protein S in the presence of calcium. J Biol Chem 1990; 265: 16082–7.

19. Dahlbäck B. Inhibition of protein Ca cofactor function of human and bovine protein S by C4b-binding protein. J Biol Chem 1986; 261: 12022–7.

20. Comp PC, Nixon RR, Cooper MR, Esmon CT. Familial protein S deficiency is associated with recurrent thrombosis. J Clin Invest 1984; 74: 2082–8.

21. Schwalbe R, Dahlbäck B, Hillarp A, Nelsestuen G. Assembly of protein S and C4b-binding protein on membranes. J Biol Chem 1990; 265: 16074–81.

22. Bertina RM, van Wijngaarden A, Reinalda-Poot J, Poort SR, Bom VJJ. Determination of plasma protein S – the protein cofactor of activated protein C. Thromb Haemostas 1985; 33: 268–72.

23. Hillarp A, Dahlbäck B. Novel subunit in C4b-binding protein required for protein S binding. J Biol Chem 1988; 263: 12759–64.

24. Makasandana C, Suvatte V, Chuansumrit A, Marlar RA, Manco Johnson MJ, Jacobson LJ, Hathaway WE. Homozygous protein S deficiency in an infant with purpura fulminans. J Pediat 1990; 117: 750–3.

25. Marlar RA, Neumann A. Neonatal purpura fulminans due to homozygous protein C or protein S deficiencies. Sem Thromb 1990; 16: 299–309.

26. Comp PC, Esmon CT. Recurrent venous thrombo-embolism in patients with a partial deficiency of protein S. N Engl J Med 1984; 311: 1525–8.

27. Schwarz HP, Fischer M, Hopmeyer P, Batard MA, Griffin JH. Plasma protein S deficiency in familial thrombotic disease. Blood 1984; 64: 1297–300.

28. Engesser L, Broekmans AW, Briët E, Brommer EJP, Bertina RM. Hereditary protein S deficiency: clinical manifestations. Ann Intern Med 1987; 106: 677–82.

29. Allaart CF, Aronson DC, Ruys Th, Rosendaal FR, van Bockel JF, Bertina RM, Briët E. Hereditary protein S deficiency in young adults with arterial occlusive disease. Thromb Haemostas 1990; 64: 206–10.

30. Sacco RL, Owen J, Mohr JR, Tatemichi Th, Grossman BA. Free protein S deficiency: a possible association with cerebrovascular occlusion. Stroke 1990; 20: 1657–61.

31. Bertina RM. Hereditary deficiencies of protein C and protein S. In: Aznar J, Espana F, eds. Protein C pathway. Iberica: Springer-Verlag, 1991; 111–20.

32. Ploos van Amstel JK, Huisman MV, Reitsma PH, Ten Cate JW, Bertina RM. Partial protein S gene deletion in a family with hereditary thrombophilia. Blood 1989; 73: 479–83.

33. Mannucci PM, Valsecchi C, Krachmalnicoff A, Faioni EM, Tripodi A. Familial dysfunction of protein S. Thromb Haemostas 1989; 62: 763–6.

34. Comp PC, Doray D, Patton D, Esmon CT. An abnormal plasma distribution of protein S occurs in functional protein S deficiency. Blood 1986; 67: 504–8.

35. Takahashi H, Tatewaki H, Wada K, Shibatu A. Plasma protein S in disseminated intravascular coagulation, liver disease, collagen disease, diabetes mellitus, and under oral anticoagulant therapy. Clin Chim Acta 1989; 182: 195–208.

36. Malm J, Laurell M, Dahlbäck B. Changes in the plasma levels of vitamin K-dependent proteins C and S and of C4b-binding protein during pregnancy and oral contraception. Br J Haematol 1988; 68: 437–43.

37. Comp PC, Thurnau GR, Webb J, Esmon CT. Functional and immunologic protein S levels are decreased during pregnancy. Blood 1986; 68: 881–5.

38. Boerger IM, Morris PC, Thurnau CT, Esmon CT, Comp PC. Oral contraceptives and gender affect protein S status. Blood 1987; 69: 692–4.

39. Schwarz HP, Schernthaner G, Griffin JH. Decreased plasma levels of protein S in well-controlled type I diabetes mellitus. Thromb Haemostas 1987; 57: 240.

40. Rostoker G, Goualt-Heilmann M, Levent M, Robeva R, Lang P, Lagrue G. High level of protein C and protein S in nephrotic syndrome. Nephron 1987; 46: 220–1.

41. Vigano d'Angelo S, D'Angelo A, Kaufman CE Jr, Sholer C, Esmon CT, Comp PC. Protein S deficiency occurs in the nephrotic syndrome. Ann Intern Med 1987; 107: 42–7.
42. Toulon P, Gaudrille S, Vitoux JF, Fiessinger JN, Sultan Y, Aiach M. High total and free protein S antigen in patients with acute deep vein thrombosis. Thromb Res 1990; 59: 213–17.
43. Kamiya T, Sugihara T, Ogata K, Saito H, Suzuki K, Nishioka J, Hashimoto S, Yamagata K. Inherited deficiency of protein S in a Japanese family with recurrent venous thrombosis: a study of three generations. Blood 1986; 67: 406–10.
44. Suzuki K, Nishioka J. Plasma protein S activity measured using Protac, a snake venom derived activator of protein C. Thromb Res 1988; 49: 241–51.
45. Wiesel ML, Charmantier JL, Freyssinet JM, Grunebaum L, Schuhler S, Cazenave JP. Screening of protein S deficiency using a functional assay. Thromb Res 1990; 58: 461–8.
46. Han P, Pradham M. A simple functional protein S assay using Protac. Clin Lab Haematol 1990; 12: 201–8.
47. Poort SR, Deutz-Terlouw PP, van Wijngaarden A, Bertina RM. Immunoradiometric assay for the calcium-stabilized conformation of human protein S. Thromb Haemostas 1987; 58: 998–1004.
48. Deutz-Terlouw PP, Ballering L, Van Wijngaarden A, Bertina RM. Two ELISAs for measurement of protein S, and their use in the laboratory diagnosis of protein S deficiency. Clin Chim Acta 1989; 186: 321–34.
49. Woodhams BJ. The simultaneous measurement of total and free protein S by ELISA. Thromb Res 1988; 50: 213–20.
50. Amiral J, Adam M, Plassant V, Minard F, Vissac AM. Immunoassays for the measurement of protein S. In: Gaffney PJ, ed. Fibrinolysis, current prospects. John Libbey, London, 1988; 125–8.
51. Krachmalnicoff A, Tombesi S, Valsecchi C, Albertini A, Mannucci PM. A monoclonal antibody to human protein S used as the capture antibody for measuring total protein S by enzyme immunoassay. Clin Chim Acta 1990; 36: 43–6.
52. Fair DS, Revak DJ. Quantitation of human protein S in the plasma of normal and warfarin treated individuals by radioimmunoassay. Thromb Res 1984; 36: 527–35.
53. Malm J, Bernhager R, Holmberg L, Dahlbäck B. Plasma concentrations of C4b-binding protein and vitamin K-dependent protein S in term and preterm infants: low levels of protein S-C4b-binding protein complexes. Br J Haematol 1988; 68: 445–9.
54. Dahlbäck B. Purification of human vitamin K-dependent protein S and its limited proteolysis by thrombin. Biochem J 1983; 209: 837–46.
55. Carlsson J, Orevin H, Axen R. Protein thiolation and reversible protein–protein conjugation. N-succinimidyl 3-(2-pyridyldithio) propionate, a new hetero-bifunctional reagent. Biochem J 1978; 173: 723–37.

13
Fibrinopeptide A (FPA)

A. HAEBERLI

INTRODUCTION

Fibrinopeptide A (FPA) is of particular interest, because it is released whenever thrombin converts fibrinogen to fibrin. Human FPA is a 16 amino acid peptide with a molecular weight of 1540, and it is cleaved from the N-terminal part of the Aα-chain of fibrinogen. Since the fibrinogen molecule has a dimer structure, two identical FPA molecules are cleaved from each fibrinogen molecule[1].

PATHOPHYSIOLOGY

Any increased FPA concentration in plasma represents thrombin activity and thus activation of the coagulation. Since with the determination of FPA a product of the last step of the coagulation cascade is measured, it may give an overall evaluation of the activation of blood coagulation.

The measurement of FPA by radioimmunoassay has been introduced by Nossel and co-workers[2,3]. Since that time it has been widely used and it is considered by many authors as an important and significant test for the diagnosis of prethrombotic and thrombotic states[4-6].

The major diagnostic applications so far are the detection of acute deep venous thrombosis[7-11], disseminated intravascular coagulation[8,12,13], pulmonary thrombosis and lung embolism[10,14], angina and myocardial infarction[15-25], cerebral infarction[26] and for the monitoring of anticoagulant therapy[18,21,27-29].

The determination of FPA has also been used to follow activation of the coagulation in cancer[30-35], during pregnancy[36], in diabetes[37-40], in liver cirrhosis[41,42] and during intake of oral contraceptives or oestrogen therapy[43-46].

METHOD OF ASSAY

Since normal concentrations are below 2 ng/ml (< 1.3 nmol/L) and pathological values very often in the range of 3–20 ng/ml (2–13 nmol/L), the only sufficiently sensitive methods are radioimmunoassay (RIA) or the enzyme-linked immunoassay (ELISA).

Nossel and co-workers were the first to develop a RIA for the determination of FPA[2,3]. The antibodies used by Nossel became available to a broader community and therefore the number of publications studying thrombotic and prethrombotic activities in different diseases by means of FPA measurements increased enormously. Since 1971 several modifications of the original RIA of Nossel have been published (e.g. refs 47 and 48). Some of these modifications have been introduced in the two RIA procedures recommended below.

Two commercial RIA kits have been available for many years. The RIA-mat FPA, originally manufactured by Mallinckrodt, now prepared and sold by Byk-Sangtec (Dietzenbach, Germany) is a ready-to-use kit with all reagents including the ^{125}I-labelled Tyr-FPA. Because of its ease of manipulation it has been used in the multicentre study on Angina Pectoris of the European Community (ECAT).

The other one is prepared by Imco (Stockholm, Sweden). It supplies only three vials containing anti-FPA antiserum, FPA-standard and Tyr-FPA for iodination with ^{125}I. The iodination of Tyr-FPA, all dilutions of the standards and the antiserum, as well as all the solutions necessary for the performance of the RIA, have to be prepared.

In 1980 a solid-phase enzyme-linked immunosorbent assay (ELISA) for the measurement of FPA was published[49]. This ELISA test is commercially available as a complete kit supplied by Stago Diagnostica (Asnières, France). Although easy to perform, it has not become as widely used as the RIA. The ELISA will not be further discussed here.

PRINCIPLE AND ASSAY CHARACTERISTICS OF THE FPA RIA

All FPA radioimmunoassays are competitive binding assays. They are based on a competition between unlabelled FPA (standard or unknown) and the ^{125}I-labelled Tyr-FPA (= tracer) for the limited amount of antibody binding sites. Tyr-FPA must be used for iodination since human FPA does not contain any tyrosine residue. As the concentration of unlabelled FPA increases, less of the tracer will be bound to the antibody. After the antibody–antigen binding reaction has been allowed to take place, free and antibody-bound FPA are separated either by charcoal adsorption of the free FPA, or by precipitating the antigen–antibody complexes with a second antibody (anti-rabbit IgG). The precipitation of the antigen–antibody complexes is performed either by the addition of polyethylene glycol to the second antibody solution (Byk-Sangtec) or with an immobilized second antibody (e.g. Immunobead Second Antibody, goat–anti-rabbit IgG, BioRad Laboratories).

The radioactivity in the supernatant representing FPA–anti-FPA complexes (charcoal system) or the radioactivity in the pellet representing FPA–anti-FPA–anti-IgG complexes (second antibody system) is counted. The standard curve is drawn by plotting the percentage of tracer bound in each standard versus its concentration on a semi-log or logit–log scale. The FPA concentration in the unknown sample is determined by comparison of the percentage of labelled FPA bound to the standard curve.

PRECAUTIONS

Although the determination of FPA is an interesting method to document activation of the coagulation with the formation of fibrin, the method has several important biological and methodological disadvantages which should be considered:

1. The biological half-life of FPA[3] is in the order of 3–5 min. Therefore any determination of the FPA concentration represents only the activity of a short time interval. Several authors have tried to overcome this problem with the determination of the FPA concentration in urine samples and thereby to obtain an estimate of the activation over a longer time period[50-53].
2. The collection of blood and the anticoagulant used are extremely important. Any incorrect procedure may easily lead to falsely elevated FPA concentrations.
3. Most antibodies used so far for the FPA determination are also reacting with the N-terminal sequence of the Aα-chains of the intact fibrinogen molecule, and thus giving rise to falsely elevated FPA values. For this reason fibrinogen must be removed completely from the plasma before the determination of FPA can be performed.

Blood sampling and processing

Blood is collected by flawless venipuncture through a 21-gauge needle at a stasis of 50 mmHg into a syringe or an evacuated tube (e.g. Vacutainer) or by dripping into an open tube, containing the anticoagulant solution. Artificially elevated FPA values may easily occur after rough or repeated venipuncture, or if the blood is not immediately mixed with the anticoagulant. Two anticoagulant solutions for the blood collection are recommended:

1. Anticoagulant solution included in the RIA-mat FPA (Byk-Sangtec). For the preparation of this anticoagulant the manufacturers' instructions must be followed. The solution may be stored at 2–8 °C for 2 months. With the use of this anticoagulant the collection of blood is only made into evacuated tubes or by dripping into open tubes containing the anticoagulant. Collection with syringes containing the potentially hazardous anticoagulant is strictly forbidden.

2. Heparin–aprotinin anticoagulant. Heparin (e.g. Liquemin, Roche) and aprotinin (e.g. Trasylol, Bayer) are dissolved in 0.9% sterile NaCl to a final concentration of 1000 U heparin and 1000 U aprotinin per ml of anticoagulant. An 0.5 ml aliquot of this anticoagulant is used for the collection of 4.5 ml of blood. With the use of this anticoagulant blood can easily be collected, without any risk, into 5 ml syringes containing the anticoagulant.

It is important that the blood is mixed quickly and thoroughly with the anticoagulant and cooled immediately to 4 °C in an ice-bath. The plasma is separated by centrifugation at 2000 g for 20 min at 2–4 °C within 1 h after collection. If not assayed immediately, the plasma samples must be stored frozen at −20 °C, or preferably at lower temperature.

Removal of fibrinogen from plasma

Unfortunately the anti-FPA antibodies supplied by Byk-Sangtec and Imco react to some extent (2–5%) with the N-terminal sequence of the Aα-chains of intact fibrinogen, thus giving rise to erroneously high FPA values. Therefore fibrinogen has to be removed from the plasma samples as completely as possible.

The adsorption of fibrinogen with bentonite has proved to be a satisfactory method. This procedure was originally introduced by Kockum and Frebelius[48]. It is the method used in the RIA-mat FPA by Byk-Sangtec and also recommended in the Imco FPA RIA procedure. In our experience it is the best method to eliminate fibrinogen almost quantitatively from plasma. It is very reproducible and the recovery of FPA is 90% and more. It is highly recommendable. It should be noted that the bentonite adsorption of fibrinogen performs well only with plasma, and not with aqueous fibrinogen solutions.

RIA-mat FPA® (BYK-SANGTEC)

Because of its ease of use this kit is highly recommended for laboratories not very familiar with radioimmunoassays. All reagents are supplied with the kit. The time to perform the assay is in the order of 3–4 h. With one kit 39 plasma samples in duplicate, including the standard curve, non-specific binding, maximal binding, control A (low FPA conc.), control B (high FPA conc.) and an in-house control plasma (all in duplicate) can be determined.

The assay is carried out strictly according to the protocol given in the instruction manual included with each kit. The controls A and B, included in the kit, must be determined in each run. In addition it is highly recommended for each laboratory to prepare its own plasma pool using either one of the anticoagulant solutions described earlier. Aliquots of this pool plasma are stored at −20 °C or lower. One aliquot of this pool should be included in each run as a control of the overall RIA quality, as well as control for the completeness of the bentonite adsorption of fibrinogen. The intra- and interassay variance is low (3–6%, 4–10% respectively).

FPA RIA Imco

For laboratories familiar with RIA methods and equipped to perform iodinations with 0.5–1.0 mCi (18.5–37 MBq), this RIA is less expensive than the ready-to-use kit RIA-mat FPA. It can easily be modified and adapted to particular needs. It is slightly more sensitive than the former RIA with a detection limit of 0.3 ng/ml as compared to 1 ng/ml.

The following modifications, as compared to the assay protocol given by Imco, have been introduced and successfully used in our laboratory for many years:

1. Bentonite adsorption of fibrinogen. The bentonite suspension is prepared exactly as described: 1 ml of the bentonite suspension is added to 0.5 ml plasma and incubated for 10 min on a rotating table at 4 °C. The mixture is then centrifuged at 2000 g and 4 °C for 20 min. The top 300 µl of the supernatant are carefully aspirated and used for the RIA. The FPA values obtained in the RIA must be corrected for the dilution caused by the bentonite adsorption step. The dilution factor has to be determined in each laboratory because of differences depending on the quality of the bentonite.

2. The standards and samples are simultaneously mixed with the tracer and the antibody and incubated at 4 °C for 16–18 h instead of the sequential incubation of the standard or sample with the antibody for 1 h, followed by the addition of the tracer with a second incubation of 30 min.

3. Separation of the free and bound tracer is performed with an immobilized second anti-rabbit IgG antibody (e.g. Immunobead Second Antibody, goat–anti-rabbit IgG, BioRad Laboratories) instead of the charcoal separation. The amount of second antibody to be added must be tested, since it is dependent on the final dilution of the anti-FPA antiserum. The incubation with the second antibody is carried out for 3 h at 4 °C on a rotating or on a rocking table. The beads are then centrifuged at 2000 g for 20 min at 4 °C, the pellet is resuspended once with 1 ml of buffer I (Imco), centrifuged again at 2000 g for 10 min. The supernatant is discarded and the pellet counted for radioactivity.

The standard curve is drawn by plotting percentage of tracer bound in each standard versus its concentration, either on logit–log paper or by any computer curve fitting program (spline function). The intra- and interassay variations are only 3–7%.

NORMAL VALUES AND QUALITY CONTROL

FPA concentrations may be expressed as ng/ml or nmol/L. To convert ng/ml to nmol/L the value in ng/ml is divided by the factor of 1.54 (e.g. 8 ng/ml:1.54 = 5.2 nmol/L).

Normal FPA concentrations are always below 2 ng/ml (< 1.3 nmol/L) and are independent of age and sex of the subject. Note: women on oral contraceptive drug treatment have elevated FPA values[44,45].

The normal FPA values should be established in every laboratory performing FPA determinations, because of the problems which may occur during blood sampling or blood processing. The collection of blood from 15–20 normal healthy control subjects may help to assure the quality of blood collection and processing, including the completeness of the elimination of fibrinogen by bentonite. Values higher than 2 ng/ml found in healthy control persons most probably point to difficulties in blood sampling, blood processing or fibrinogen adsorption, provided the RIA is adequately performed. The latter may easily be controlled by intra-assay control samples (e.g. control A and B in the RIA-mat FPA).

PERSPECTIVES

Recently Kudryk and co-workers have presented an FPA-ELISA using a monoclonal antibody which does not react with the N-terminal part of the Aα-chain of intact fibrinogen, and which is specific for free FPA[54]. Therefore the presence of fibrinogen in the plasma does not give rise to elevated FPA values. This allows omission of the tedious removal of fibrinogen before the assay. Unfortunately with a detection limit of 45 ng/ml, or 30 nmol/L, the ELISA is not yet sufficiently sensitive to be used in most clinical situations. It is certainly in this direction that improvements of an immunological FPA assay should be attempted.

References

1. Marder VJ, Francis CW, Doolittle RF. Fibrinogen, structure and physiology. In: Colman RW, Hirsh J, Marder VJ, Salzman EW (eds), Haemostasis and thrombosis. Philadelphia: Lippincott, 1982; 145–63.
2. Nossel HL, Younger LR, Wilner GD, Procupez D, Canfield RE, Butler VP. Radioimmunoassay of human fibrinopeptide A. Proc Natl Acad Sci USA 1971; 68: 2350–3.
3. Nossel HL, Yudelman I, Canfield RE, Butler VP, Spanondis K, Wilner GD, Qureshi GD. Measurement of fibrinopeptide A in human blood. J Clin Invest 1974; 54: 43–53.
4. Bauer KA, Rosenberg RD. The pathophysiology of the prethrombotic state in humans: Insights gained from studies using markers of hemostatic system activation. Blood 1987; 70: 343–50.
5. Hirsh J. Blood tests for the diagnosis of venous and arterial thrombosis. Blood 1981; 57: 1–8.
6. Joist JH. Fibrinopeptide A in the diagnosis and treatment of deep venous thrombosis and pulmonary embolism. Clin Lab Med 1984; 4: 363–80.
7. Douglas JT, Blamey SL, Lowe GDO, Carter DC, Forbes CD. Plasma beta-thromboglobulin, fibrinopeptide A and Bβ 15 – 42 antigen in relation to postoperative DVT, malignancy and stanozolol treatment. Thromb Haemostas 1985; 53: 235–8.
8. Leeksma OC, Meijer-Huizinga F, Stoepman-van-Dalen EA, van Ginkel CJW, van Aken WG, van Mourik JA. Fibrinopeptide A and the phosphate content of fibrinogen in venous thromboembolism and disseminated intravascular coagulation. Blood 1986; 67: 1460–7.
9. Nossel HL. Radioimmunoassay of fibrinopeptides in relation to intravascular coagulation and thrombosis. N Engl J Med 1976; 295: 428–32.

FIBRINOPEPTIDE A (FPA)

10. Van Hulsteijn H, Briet E, Koch C, Hermans J, Bertina R. Diagnostic value of fibrinopeptide A and beta-thromboglobulin in acute deep venous thrombosis and pulmonary embolism. Acta Med Scand 1982; 211: 323–30.
11. Yudelman IM, Nossel HL, Kaplan KL, Hirsh J. Plasma fibrinopeptide A levels in symptomatic venous thromboembolism. Blood 1978; 51: 1189–95.
12. Cronlund M, Hardin J, Burton J, Lee L, Haber E, Bloch KJ. Fibrinopeptide A in plasma of normal subjects and patients with disseminated intravascular coagulation and systemic lupus erythematosus. J Clin Invest 1976; 58: 142–51.
13. Mombelli G, Monotti R, Haeberli A, Straub PW. Relationship between fibrinopeptide A and fibrinogen/fibrin fragment E in thromboembolism, DIC and various non-thromboembolic diseases. Thromb Haemostas 1987; 58: 758–63.
14. Eisenberg PR, Lucore C, Kaufman L, Sobel BE, Jaffe AS, Rich S. Fibrinopeptide A levels indicative of pulmonary vascular thrombosis in patients with primary pulmonary hypertension. Circulation 1990; 82: 841–7.
15. Douglas JT, Lowe GDO, Forbes CD, Prentice CRM. Plasma fibrinopeptide A and beta-thromboglobulin in patients with chest pain. Thromb Haemostas 1983; 50: 541–2.
16. Eisenberg PR, Sherman LA, Schectman K, Perez J, Sobel BE, Jaffe AS. Fibrinopeptide A: a marker of acute coronary thrombosis. Circulation 1985; 71: 912–18.
17. Gallino A, Haeberli A, Baur HR, Straub PW. Fibrin formation and platelet aggregation in patients with severe coronary artery disease: relationship with the degree of myocardial ischemia. Circulation 1985; 72: 27–30.
18. Gallino A, Haeberli A, Hess T, Mombelli G, Straub PW. Fibrin formation and platelet aggregation in patients with acute myocardial infarction: effects of intravenous and subcutaneous low-dose heparin. Am Heart J 1986; 112: 285–90.
19. Gensini GF, Rostagno C, Abbate R, Favilla S, Mannucci PM, Neri Serneri GG. Increased protein C and fibrinopeptide A concentration in patients with angina. Thromb Res 1988; 50: 517–25.
20. Irie T, Imaaizumi T, Matuguchi T, Koyanagi S, Kanaide H, Takeshita A, Nakamura M. Increased fibrinopeptide A during anginal attacks in patients with variant angina. J Am Coll Cardiol 1989; 14: 589–94.
21. Mombelli G, Im Hof V, Haeberli A, Straub PW. Effect of heparin on plasma fibrinopeptide A (fpA) in acute myocardial infarction. Circulation 1984; 69: 684–9.
22. Neri Serneri G, Gensini GF, Carnovali M, Prisco D, Rogasi PG, Casolo GC, Fazi A, Abbate R. Association between time of increased fibrinopeptide A levels in plasma and episodes of spontaneous angina: A controlled prospective study. Am Heart J 1987; 113: 672–8.
23. Nichols AB, Owen J, Kaplan KL, Sciacca RR, Cannon PJ, Nossel HL. Fibrinopeptide A, platelet factor 4, and β-thromboglobulin levels in coronary heart disease. Blood 1982; 60: 650–4.
24. Théroux P, Latour JG, Leger-Gauthier C, De Lara J. Fibrinopeptide A and platelet factor levels in unstable angina pectoris. Circulation 1987; 75: 156–62.
25. Van Hulsteijn H, Kolff J, Briet E, van der Laarse A, Bertina R. Fibrinopeptide A and beta-thromboglobulin in patients with angina pectoris and acute myocardial infarction. Am Heart J 1984; 107: 39–45.
26. Landi G, Barbarotto R, Morabito A, D'Angelo A, Mannucci PM. Prognostic significance of fibrinopeptide A in survivors of cerebral infarction. Stroke 1990; 21: 424–7.
27. Conway EM, Bauer KA, Barzegar S, Rosenberg RD. Suppression of hemostatic system activation by oral anticoagulants in the blood of patients with thrombotic diseases. J Clin Invest 1987; 80: 1535–44.
28. Peuscher FW, van Aken WG, Flier OThN, Stoepman-van Dalen EA, Cremer-Goote TM, van Mourik JA. Effect of anticoagulant treatment measured by fibrinopeptide A (fpA) in patients with venous thromboembolism. Thromb Res 1980; 18: 33–43.
29. Yudelman I, Greenberg J. Factors affecting fibrinopeptide A levels in patients with venous thromboembolism during anticoagulant therapy. Blood 1982; 59: 787–92.
30. Auger MJ, Galloway MJ, Leinster SJ, McVerry BA, Mackie MJ. Elevated fibrinopeptide A levels in patients with clinically localised breast carcinoma. Haemostasis 1987; 17: 336–9.
31. Edwards RL, Klaus M, Matthews E, McCullen C, Bona RD, Rickles FR. Heparin abolishes the chemotherapy-induced increase in plasma fibrinopeptide A levels. Am J Med 1990; 89: 25–8.
32. Gugliotta L, Vigano S, D'Angelo A, Guarini A, Tura S, Mannucci PM. High fibrinopeptide A (FPA) levels in acute non-lymphocytic leukemia are reduced by heparin administration.

Thromb Haemostas 1984; 52: 301–4.

33. Mombelli G, Roux A, Haeberli A, Straub PW. Comparison of ^{125}I-fibrinogen kinetics and fibrinopeptide A in patients with disseminated neoplasias. Blood 1982; 60: 381–8.

34. Myers TJ, Rickles FR, Barb C, Cronlund M. Fibrinopeptide A in acute leukemia: Relationship of activation of blood coagulation to disease activity. Blood 1981; 57: 518–25.

35. Peuscher FW, Cleton FJ, Armstrong L, Stoepman-van-Dalen EA, van Mourik JA, van Aken WG. Significance of plasma fibrinopeptide A (fpA) in patients with malignancy. J Lab Clin Med 1980; 96: 5–14.

36. Douglas JT, Shah M, Lowe GDO, Belah JJF, Forbes CD, Prentice CRM. Plasma fibrinopeptide A and β-thromboglobulin in preeclampsia and pregnancy hypertension. Thromb Haemostas 1982; 47: 54–8.

37. Jones RL. Fibrinopeptide A in diabetes mellitus. Relation to levels of blood glucose, fibrinogen disappearance and hemodynamic changes. Diabetes 1985; 34: 836–43.

38. Librenti MC, D'Angelo A, Micossi P, Garimberti B, Mannucci PM, Pozza G. β-thromboglobulin and fibrinopeptide A in diabetes mellitus as markers of vascular damage. Acta Diabetol Lat 1985; 22: 39–45.

39. Rosove MH, Frank HJL, Harwig SSL. Plasma β-thromboglobulin, platelet factor 4, fibrinopeptide A, and other hemostatic functions during improved, short-term glycemic control in diabetes mellitus. Diabetes Care 1984; 7: 174–9.

40. Roy MS, Podgar MJ, Rick ME. Plasma fibrinopeptide A, β-thromboglobulin, and platelet factor 4 in diabetic retinopathy. Invest Opthalmol Vis Sci 1988; 29: 856–60.

41. Coccheri S, Mannucci PM, Palaretti G, Gervasoni W, Poggi M, Vigano S. Significance of plasma fibrinopeptide A and high molecular weight fibrinogen in patients with liver cirrhosis. Br J Haematol 1982; 52: 503–9.

42. Marongiu F, Mameli G, Acca MR, Mulas G, Medda A, Tronci MB, Mamusa AM, Balestrieri A. Fibrinopeptide A and Bβ 15-42 in liver cirrhosis. Haemostasis 1988; 18: 126–28.

43. Alkjaersig N, Fletcher AP, de Ziegler D, Steingold KA, Meldrum DR, Judd HL. Blood coagulation in postmenopausal women given oestrogen treatment: comparison of transdermal and oral administration. J Lab Clin Med 1988; 111: 224–8.

44. Inauen W, Baumgartner HR, Haeberli A, Straub PW. Excessive deposition of fibrin, platelets and platelet thrombi on vascular subendothelium during contraceptive drug treatment. Thromb Haemostas 1987; 57: 306–9.

45. Melis GB, Fruzzetti F, Paoletti AM, Carmassi F, Fioretti P. Fibrinopeptide A plasma levels during low-estrogen oral contraceptive treatment. Contraception 1984; 30: 575–83.

46. Melis GB, Fruzzetti F, Ricci C, Carmassi F, Fioretti P. Oral contraceptives and venous thromboembolic disease: the effect of the oestrogen dose. Maturitas, Suppl. 1988; 1: 131–9.

47. Hofmann V, Straub PW. A radioimmunoassay technique for the rapid measurement of human fibrinopeptide A. Thromb Res 1977; 11: 171–81.

48. Kockum C, Frebelius S. Rapid radioimmunoassay of human fibrinopeptide A – removal of cross-reacting fibrinogen with bentonite. Thromb Res 1980; 19: 589–98.

49. Soria J, Soria C, Ryckewaert JJ. A solid phase immuno enzymological assay for the measurement of human fibrinopeptide A. Thromb Res 1980; 20: 425–35.

50. Alkjaersig N, Fletcher AP. Catabolism and excretion of fibrinopeptide A. Blood 1982; 60: 148–56.

51. Gallino A, Haeberli A, Straub PW. Fibrinopeptide A excretion in urine in patients with atherosclerotic artery disease. Thromb Res 1985; 38: 237–44.

52. Leeksma OC, Meijer-Huizinga F, Stoepman-van Dalen EA, van Aken WG, van Mourik JA. Fibrinopeptide A in urine from patients with venous thromboembolism, disseminated intravascular coagulation and rheumatoid arthritis – Evidence for dephosphorylation and carboxyterminal degradation of the peptide by the kidney. Thromb Haemostas 1985; 54: 792–8.

53. Wilensky RL, Zeller JA, Wish M, Tulchinsky M. Urinary fibrinopeptide A levels in ischemic heart disease. J Am Coll Cardiol 1989; 14: 597–603.

54. Kudryk B, Gidlund M, Rohoza A, Ahadi M, Coiffe D, Weitz JI. Use of a synthetic homologue of human fibrinopeptide A for production of a monoclonal antibody specific for the free peptide. Blood 1989; 74: 1036–44.

14
Thrombin–antithrombin III complexes

J. HARENBERG

INTRODUCTION

Blood coagulation terminates by the activation of prothrombin to thrombin and subsequent conversion of fibrinogen to fibrin. During these processes various activation peptides are released. Fragments F_{1+2} are split off from prothrombin by the prothrombokinase complex. Specific immunoassays have been developed to determine the concentration of these peptides in plasma.

Antithrombin III is an α_2-globulin with a molecular weight of about 65 000 and is synthesized in the liver. Thrombin is released by activation of the proenzyme prothrombin. Antithrombin III inhibits thrombin by forming an inactive protein/inhibitor complex[1,2].

Thrombin is inhibited by antithrombin III, forming a thrombin–antithrombin III (TAT) complex. Therefore the TAT complex should also reflect the functional state of the coagulation system. This complex is influenced to a smaller degree by external influences like the technique of blood sampling. Therefore TAT has been adopted in a large set of clinical investigations and represents a diagnostic tool for the detection of hypercoagulability.

METHODS OF ASSAY

Principle and assay characteristics

The assay principle was described first by Neumann et al.[3] and Brower et al.[4] for the detection of elastase–α_1-antitrypsin complexes and is based on the properties of the appropriate antibodies to bind selectively the corresponding moieties of the complex. Thus the assay for measuring the TAT complex consists of antibodies directed against thrombin as well as antithrombin III. Nanogram quantities of TAT can be detected by these assays. Prothrombin, as well as antithrombin III, are not detected by the antibodies.

The TAT complex has a molecular weight of 88 000 and elutes as a single peak from a sodium dodecyl sulphate gel[5].

Materials

At present only one enzyme immunoassay test kit is commercially available. This ELISA test system has been developed by Behring Werke AG, Marburg, Germany[6] and contains:

1. Plastic tubes coated with antibodies to human thrombin, stability 4 weeks at $+4\,°C$;
2. antibodies to human antithrombin III conjugated to horse–rabbit peroxidase (preservative phenol max 1 g/l), stability 4 weeks at $+4\,°C$ or 3 months at $-20\,°C$;
3. buffered solution containing rabbit γ-globulin and 5 mg/ml bovine serum albumin (preservative phenol max 1 g/l), stability 4 weeks at $+4\,°C$ or 3 months at $-20\,°C$;
4. buffered solution for dilution of plasma samples 0.1 mol Tris-HCl pH 7.4 with 5 mg/ml bovine serum albumin (preservative sodium azide max 1 g/L), stability 4 weeks at $+4\,°C$ or 3 months at $-20\,°C$;
5. PBS phosphate buffer saline solution containing 0.01% Tween, stability as given on the vial;
6. citrate buffer solution containing 0.1 mol/L citrate and 0.2 mol/L sodium phosphate, pH 7.0 (preservative sodium-p-ethyl-mercury-mercapto-benzene sulphonate max 0.1 g/L);
7. 200 mg/ml 1,2-phenylenediamine monohydrochloride, stability only in the dark and 3 h at $+4\,°C$;
8. 0.5 N sulphuric acid, stability as given on the vial.

Procedure

Venous blood is withdrawn from patients, in plastic syringes or siliconized glass tubes containing 3.8% sodium citrate (9:1, v/v). Samples are centrifuged for 15 min at 2000 g and at $+4\,°C$ and obtained plasma is immediately shock-frozen and stored at $-30\,°C$.

The antibody specific to thrombin is bound to polystyrene plastic tubes. The tubes contain a volume of 2.0 ml or 0.35 ml on microtitre plates. Plasma is incubated in the test tube. The thrombin of the TAT complex reacts with the thrombin antibody on the surface of the plastic tube. The antithrombin III antibody is conjugated with peroxidase. This antibody reacts with the antithrombin moiety of the TAT complex which was bound to the thrombin antibody on the surface of the plastic tube. After washing the samples with buffer o-phenyldiamine hydrochloride is added to the plasma sample and thereafter hydrogen peroxide is added to the test tube. The reaction of the release of o-phenyldiamine is stopped by adding H_2SO_4 and absorbance is read at 492 nm.

118

Evaluation of results

Thrombosis and pulmonary embolism

Patients with deep vein thrombosis (DVT) and/or pulmonary embolism have been studied to demonstrate the validity of the TAT assay. Elevated plasma concentrations have been found in all patients with very recent clinical symptoms[7]. During heparin treatment TAT levels decrease in patients with pulmonary embolism or DVT[8]. The diagnostic value of TAT has been quantitated in outpatients with suspected DVT based on clinical symptoms. The sensitivity for the detection of DVT was 37% and the specificity was 88% using this assay[9]. Other fibrinogen degradation products have also been determined in this study. All assays proved to be of little value in outpatients for detection of DVT, due to the low sensitivity.

Postoperative care

TAT complexes have been measured in postoperative care medicine with the aim of defining a predictive index for the development of DVT. TAT levels were significantly higher in patients developing DVT when compared to patients without DVT. Statistical analysis revealed no satisfactory discriminative power for the diagnosis of developing DVT at any of the studied cut-off values for TAT[10]. TAT levels were measured in plasma of patients who underwent total knee replacement in order to determine the possible value of this assay in screening for thromboembolic complications. No difference was observed in patients who developed DVT and those who did not. However, the number of patients was too small to draw definite conclusions from these data[11]. In summary the data do not yet give sufficient information on the value of predictivity of DVT using the TAT assay, due to the small number of patients and positive events.

Myocardial infarction and angina pectoris

In patients with acute uncomplicated myocardial infarction and with unstable angina pectoris elevated plasma levels of TAT were found[12]. Low-dose heparin significantly reduces the rise of TAT complexes after myocardial infarction[13]. Elevated plasma levels in patients with coronary heart disease were also found by others. These levels increased after a standardized exercise in these patients as well as in healthy controls, indicating that patients with coronary heart disease possess a latent hypercoagulable state[14]. However, no differences of TAT levels were found in patients with angina pectoris who developed myocardial infarction compared to a healthy control group[15]. In patients with successful thrombolysis of an occluded coronary vessel TAT levels decreased to the normal range whereas in patients with no successful thrombolysis TAT levels remained unchanged or increased[16].

119

Disseminated intravascular coagulation and liver disease

Diseases with disseminated intravascular coagulation may also be related to elevated levels of TAT. The sensitivity of the TAT levels is higher for detection of disseminated intravascular coagulation than for myocardial infarction[17,18]. In patients with liver disease plasma levels of TAT were elevated, indicating an activation of the coagulation system[19]. The plasmin−α_2-antiplasmin (PAP) complexes are also increased in patients with liver disease. Therefore ratios were calculated to determine which effect of the two systems is more important. Patients with sepsis and decompensated liver disease showed the highest TAT/PAP ratio[20].

Malignancy, leukaemia and chemotherapy

TAT concentrations were investigated in patients with malignant diseases in order to obtain information on activation of the coagulation system[21]. Detailed studies indicated that TAT levels are significantly higher in patients with disseminated malignancy than in patients with limited disease. This indicates a state of definite hypercoagulation in these diseases[22]. Activation of blood coagulation has been described in patients with acute promyelocytic leukaemia due to increased TAT levels[23]. Treatment of patients with acute promyelocytic leukaemia with L-asparaginase resulted in a further elevation of TAT complexes. Patients who received antithrombin III concentrate supplementation did not show increases of TAT levels[24].

Diabetes mellitus

In patients with diabetes mellitus an activation of the coagulation system has been described several times in the past, and has been attributed to the morphological changes of the microvascular system. The levels of TAT were significantly elevated in diabetes mellitus as compared to a healthy control group[25]. However, this has not been supported as yet by others[26].

Thus a variety of clinical conditions has been reported to be associated with an increase of the TAT concentration (Table 14.1).

Table 14.1 Elevated concentrations of TAT in plasma in relation to pathological conditions

	Reference
Hereditary diseases	
not reported so far	
Acquired diseases	
acute deep vein thrombosis	10
acute pulmonary embolism	10
oral anticoagulation and heparinization	11, 16
postoperative medicine	13
acute myocardial infarction and angina pectoris	15, 17, 19
disseminated intravascular coagulation	20, 21
liver disease	22, 23
malignancy, leukaemia and chemotherapy	24, 25
diabetes mellitus	28

In summary, levels of TAT are elevated in acute stages of diseases whereas in subacute or chronic states of diseases contradictory results are reported. Thus it can be assumed that TAT plasma levels are of clinical significance for screening hypercoagulation in patients developing DVT or pulmonary embolism.

Difficulties, source of error

The following points may influence the validity of the results: incorrect blood sampling with coagulation of blood *in vitro* and incorrect storage of the reagents. Blood samples from patients with haemolysis, hypercholesterolaemia, hyperbilirubinaemia and high levels of rheumatic factors may influence the results.

The concentrations of TAT are influenced by technical problems during withdrawal of blood. Blood sampling has to be performed very carefully by a clean venipuncture. The tourinque of the forearm has to be released after puncture of a large vein of the forearm and free-flowing blood has to be taken into a plastic syringe or into a siliconized glass tube containing 3.8% sodium citrate. If any coagulation takes place during or after blood sampling TAT complexes are formed *in vitro*. This leads to false high concentrations of TAT in plasma.

Reference values

The concentration of TAT in plasma samples of healthy subjects is not normally distributed. Values range from 0.50 to 3.25 ng/ml with a peak at 1.25 ng/ml[27-29].

Control and calibration procedures

Standard curves are linear in a range of 0.5 to 60 ng/ml. The recovery rate of purified TAT added to normal plasma ranged from 90% to 110%. The intra-assay coefficient of variation was 2.0–6.1%. The inter-assay coefficient of variation is between 2.4% and 4.7% when 2–60 ng/ml TAT were added to pool plasma. The linearity of plasma samples containing high concentrations of TAT is good when the plasma concentrations were determined after various dilutions of the samples with TAT-poor pool plasma. The lower detection limit of the assay is 0.5 ng/ml.

The correlation between the ECAT assay and other available methods of assay

The ELISA for the determination of TAT can be performed with larger and smaller volumes of the reagents. The latter method has been developed in our laboratory on microtitre plates and is now available from Behringwerke AG. The correlation between these two techniques is $r = 0.97$. No other methods are available at the moment from other manufacturers.

References

1. Teitel JM, Bauer KA, Lau HK, Rosenberg RD. Studies of the prothrombin activation pathway utilizing radioimmunoassays for the F_2F_{1+2} fragment and thrombin–antithrombin complex. Blood 1982; 59: 1086–91.
2. Owen WG. Evidence for the formation of an ester between thrombin and heparin coafactor. Biochim Biophys Acta 1975; 405: 380–7.
3. Neumann S, Gunzer G, Hennrich N, Lang H. PMN-elastase assay: enzyme immunoassay for human polymorphonuclear elastase complexed with proteinase inhibitor. J Clin Chem Clin Biochem 1984; 22: 693.
4. Brower MS, Harpel PC. Alpha 1-antitrypsin human leukocyte elastase complexes in blood: quantification by an enzyme linked differential antibody immunosorbent assay and comparison with alpha-2-plasmin inhibitor–plasmin complexes. Blood 1983; 61: 842–9.
5. Lau HK, Rosenberg RD. The isolation and characterization of a specific antibody population directed against the thrombin–antithrombin complex. J Biol Chem 1980; 255: 5885–93.
6. Enzygnost TAT ELISA test kit. Enzyme immunoassay for the determination of thrombin/antithrombin III complex. Behringwerke AG, Marburg, Germany, 1988.
7. Blanke H, Praetorius G, Leschke M, Seitz R, Egbring R, Strauer BE. Diagnostic value of thrombin–antithrombin III complex in pulmonary embolism and in deep vein thrombosis – comparison with fibrinopeptide A, platelet factor 4, and beta-thromboglobulin. Klin Wochenschr 1987; 65: 757–63.
8. Meyer D, Tsakiris DA, Marbet GA. Thrombin–antithrombin III complexes as a measure of effective heparin treatment? Schweiz Med Wochenschr 1989; 119: 1352–4.
9. van Bergen PF, Knot EA, Jonker JJ, de Boer AC, de Maat MP. Is quantitative determination of fibrin(ogen) degradation products and thrombin–antithrombin III complexes useful to diagnose deep venous thrombosis in outpatients? Thromb Haemostas 1989; 62: 1043–5.
10. Hoek JA, Nurmohamed MT, ten Cate JW, Buller HR, Knipscheer HC. Thrombin–antithrombin III complexes in the prediction of deep vein thrombosis following total hip replacement. Thromb Haemostas 1989; 62: 1050–2.
11. de Prost D, Olliver V, Vie P, Bencerraf R, Duparc J, Khoury A. D-dimer and thrombin–antithrombin III complex levels uncorrelated with phlebographic findings in 11 total knee replacement patients. Ann Biol Clin Paris 1990; 48: 235–8.
12. Carvalho de Sous J, Azevedo J, Soria C, Barros F, Ribeiro C, Parreira F, Caen JP. Factor VII hyperactivity in acute myocardial thrombosis – a relation to the coagulation activation. Thromb Res 1988; 51: 165–73.
13. Pseja P, Lewandowski K, Turowiecka Z, Zozulinska M, Tokarz A, Zawilska K. Fluctuation of thrombin–antithrombin III complex in patients with acute myocardial infarction – influence of low-dose heparin administration. Folia Haematol Leipz 1990; 117: 219–23.
14. Uno M, Tsuji H, Watanabe M, Takada O, Kobayashi K, Takabuchi H, Shirai K, Sawada S, Toyoda T, Yamamoto K. Application of thrombin–antithrombin III complex for detecting a latent hypercoagulable state in patients with coronary artery disease. Jpn Circ J 1989; 53: 1185–91.
15. Munkvad S, Gram J, Jespersen J. A depression of active tissue plasminogen activator in plasma characterizes patients with unstable angina pectoris who develop myocardial infarction. Eur Heart J 1990; 11: 525–8.
16. Gulba DC, Daniel WG, Simon R, Jost S, Barthels M, Amende I, Rafflenbeul W, Lichtlen PR. Role of thrombolysis and thrombin in patients with acute coronary occlusion during percutaneous transluminal coronary angioplasty. J Am Coll Cardiol 1990; 16: 563–8.
17. Boisclair MD, Lane DA, Wilde JT, Ireland H, Preston FE, Ofosu FA. A comparative evaluation of assays for markers of activated coagulation and/or fibrinolysis: thrombin–antithrombin complex, D-dimer and fibrinogen/fibrin fragment E antigen. Br J Haematol 1990; 74: 471–9.
18. Seitz R, Egbring R, Wagner C, Dati F. Thrombin–antithrombin III complex (TAT): a marker for activation of intravascular coagulation. Internist 1990; 31: 69–74.
19. Takahashi H, Tatewaki W, Wada K, Yoshikawa A, Shibata A. Thrombin and plasmin generation in patients with liver disease. Am J Hematol 1989; 32: 30–5.
20. Takahashi H, Tatewaki W, Wada K, Hanano M, Shibata A. Thrombin vs plasmin generation in disseminated intravascular coagulation associated with various underlying disorders. Am

J Hematol 1990; 33: 90–5.
21. Rocha E, Paramo JA, Fernandez FJ, Cuesta B, Hernandez M, Paloma MJ, Rifon J. Clotting activation and impairment of fibrinolysis in malignancy. Thromb Res 1989; 54: 699–707.
22. Lindahl AK, Sandset PM, Abildgaard U. Indices of hypercoagulation in cancer as compared with those in acute inflammation and acute infarction. Haemostasis 1990; 20: 253–62.
23. Avvisati G, ten Cate JW, Sturk A, Lamping R, Petti MG, Mandelle F. Acquired alphas-2-antiplasmin deficiency in acute promyelocytic leukaemia. Br J Haematol 1988; 70: 43–8.
24. Gugliotta L, D'Angelo A, Mattioli Belmonte M, Vigano-D'Angelo S, Colombo G, Datani L, Gianni L, Lauria F, Tura S. Hypercoagulability during L-asparaginase treatment: the effect of antithrombin III supplementation in vivo. Br J Haematol 1990; 74: 465–70.
25. Takahashi H, Tsuda A, Tatewaki W, Wada K, Niwano H, Shibata A. Activation of blood coagulation and fibrinolysis in diabetes mellitus: evaluation by plasma levels of thrombin–antithrombin III complex and plasmin-alpha-2-plasmin inhibitor complex. Thromb Res 1989; 55: 727–35.
26. van Wersch JWJ, Westerhuis LW, Venekamp WJ. Coagulation activation in diabetes mellitus. Haemostasis 1990; 20: 263–9.
27. Pelzer H, Schwarz A, Heimburger N. Determination of human thrombin–antithrombin III complex in plasma with an enzyme linked immunosorbent assay. Thromb Haemostas 1988; 59: 101–6.
28. Heimburger N, Pelzer H. Determination of human thrombin-antithrombin III complex by enzyme immunoassay. Folia Haematol Leipz 1988; 115: 269–73.
29. Hoek JA, Sturk A, ten Cate JW, Lamping RJ, Berends F, Borm JJ. Laboratory and clinical evaluation of an assay of thrombin–antithrombin III complexes in plasma. Clin Chem 1988; 34: 2058–62.

15
Euglobulin clot lysis time

P. C. COOPER and F. E. PRESTON

PRINCIPLES AND ASSAY CHARACTERISTICS

The euglobulin clot lysis time (ECLT) has been applied as a tool for the investigation of fibrinolysis for many years. Sherry *et al.* demonstrated increased fibrinolysis as shortening of the ECLT post-exercise, adrenaline infusion, venous occlusion and following electroconvulsive therapy[1]. Kowalski *et al.* reviewed ECLT results from a number of workers and showed that their technique of euglobulin fractionation resulted in a product containing variable amounts of procoagulant proteins, all plasma plasminogen, but which contained only traces of antiplasmin activity[2].

Plasma is fractionated by dilution to a low ionic strength and is acidified in order to precipitate the euglobulin fraction, which is retained, whilst the major proportion of fibrinolytic inhibitors are discarded. The euglobulin fraction is dissolved and the fibrinogen clotted; clot lysis is then timed. This assay makes use of the patient's fibrin as substrate. The assay has been simplified by automated clot lysis detection by means of a dedicated clot lysis detector and by microplate reader[3,4].

The ECLT is a global test of fibrinolysis which can measure both baseline and stimulated fibrin dissolution in a milieu largely depleted of natural inhibitors of fibrinolysis. The ECLT is largely dependent on the activity of both tissue plasminogen activator (t-PA) and plasminogen activator–inhibitor (PAI)[5]. Increased fibrinolysis, for example excessive production of t-PA, results in a bleeding diathesis[6]; whereas a decreased level of fibrinolysis, for example due to high levels of PAI, is associated with thrombosis[7], although this association has recently been questioned[8,9].

125

MATERIALS

Plasma samples

Citrated plasma prepared according to the protocols in Chapters 1 and 2 is tested, this may be either cold fresh plasma (from blood no more than 1 h old) or snap frozen plasma (stored at $-70\,°C$) which is later thawed for 3–5 min at $37\,°C$ and then used immediately. However, we have observed that the ECLT performed on fresh plasma is consistently 10% shorter than the ECLT of the same plasma which is snap-frozen and stored at $-70\,°C$ before testing. Therefore it is recommended that plasma is either tested immediately or snap-frozen then tested later, but the techniques are not interchanged.

Distilled water

Freshly distilled water is stored in an airtight container in order to avoid acidification by carbon dioxide absorption.

Acetic acid

Glacial acetic acid (0.25% v/v) in distilled water.

Tris buffer

0.1 mol/L Tris HCl; pH to 7.5 with 0.1 mol/L sodium hydroxide; whilst mixing add 0.1% v/v Tween 80.

Calcium–thrombin solution

Bovine thrombin diluted to 20 u/ml in saline (store in aliquots at $-20\,°C$); 0.05 mol/L calcium chloride. Working solution: mix equal volumes of thrombin and calcium chloride.

PROCEDURE

1. Distilled water (1.8 ml) is added to a 75×12 mm polystyrene tube. The tube is then placed in a flask containing melting ice and left at least 10 min to cool to $0\,°C$.
2. Plasma (200 µl) is added to the cold distilled water and the tube is continually mixed as 150 µl 0.25% acetic acid is slowly added drop by drop in order to bring the pH to approximately 5.9. The use of a pH meter to titrate the amount of acetic acid to bring the pH to exactly 5.9 will result in a slightly narrower normal range as this volume varies slightly from plasma to plasma.
3. The tube is covered with parafilm and incubated on melting ice for 30 min.
4. The tubes are centrifuged for 10 min at $2100\,g$ at $4\,°C$.

5. The supernatant is decanted off and the tube drained by inversion on to filter paper for 2 min. The inside of the tube is then carefully wiped dry by means of a probe wrapped in tissue paper (taking care not to disturb the precipitate) – this is carried out twice in order to remove the maximum of the supernatant.
6. The precipitate is dissolved by adding 200 µl Tris buffer, followed by the use of a plastic 200 µl pipette to mobilize the precipitate whilst avoiding bubble formation. If difficulty is encountered in solubilization, the tube may be warmed for 30 s at 37 °C whilst mixing.
7. To one tube at a time: add 100 µl calcium–thrombin, immediately tilt four times to mix before clot formation. Place at 37 °C and note the time each tube is clotted.
8. Every 10 min, during the first hour, carefully lift the tube from the water bath (taking great care not to disturb the clot) and look for the presence of clot lysis. After 1 h observe the clot at 15-min intervals. When lysis has begun in a tube observe the clot every 5 min. Lysis is complete when no clot is visible, although sometimes small flecks of white particulate matter remain in a tube after clot lysis is complete.

EVALUATION OF RESULTS

Tissue plasminogen activator activity increases greatly during the day, resulting in a shortening of the ECLT, making it necessary to standardize the timing of blood sampling – normally between 08.30 and 10.30 a.m. Food and drink may also affect t-PA and PAI in various ways which modify the ECLT, see the recommendations on preanalytical variables in Chapter 1. The ECLT may be tested using samples taken under baseline conditions as well as in samples following *in vivo* stimulation of fibrinolysis by venous occlusion, exercise and desamino-8-D-arginine vasopressin (DDAVP). Many early reports of fibrinolytic potential are difficult to assess because of unstated patient preparation and sample processing, both of which are critical because of physiological variations and the *in vitro* lability of t-PA and PAI. It is therefore essential that the protocols described in Chapters 1 and 2 for obtaining baseline and post-venous occlusion blood specimens for fibrinolytic activity assays are followed rigidly for the ECLT.

The ECLT is shortened in conditions of increased fibrinolysis, for example following exercise or adrenaline infusion; and is prolonged in conditions with impaired fibrinolysis, for example postoperatively and in many patients with a history of thrombosis.

DIFFICULTIES, SOURCES OF ERROR AND TROUBLE-SHOOTING

Patients must be free of thrombosis for at least 3 months before being tested, and must have no infection or other acute-phase reaction at the time of venipuncture. Patients showing a prolonged ECLT must be retested at a later date to confirm that the abnormality is not due to a subclinical infection or other acute-phase process which will result in increased PAI levels and prolonged ECLT.

The importance of obtaining a valid sample cannot be over-emphasized (see Chapters 1 and 2), because of pre-analytical variables in patient selection and preparation as well as in proper sample handling.

The procedure of performing the ECLT must be standardized, particularly because of the lability of t-PA and the variables in the preparation of the euglobulin fraction. The euglobulin fraction has been reported to contain variable amounts of PAI and C1 esterase inhibitor, but virtually no α_2-antiplasmin as long as the supernatant is fully removed. In 1986 a survey performed by Dr Walker, for the task force of the British Committee for the Standardisation in Haematology, Haemostasis and Thrombosis, demonstrated that in the preparation of euglobulin fractions, plasma dilutions ranged from 1/3 to 1/20 and acidification ranged from pH < 5.0 up to pH 6.1–7.0. In the method reported here we have observed that acidification to precipitate the euglobulin fraction in 40 plasma samples resulted in a pH which varied from 5.55 to 6.25 (mean 5.89) and that there is a 20% shortening in ECLT prepared from euglobulin precipitated at pH 6.25 compared with pH 5.55, which suggests that titration of the amount of acetic acid will result in a narrowing of the observed normal range, although we do not consider this procedure to be essential. A standardized technique of patient preparation, plasma preparation and ECLT methodology should greatly aid both quality control and the understanding of results obtained from different centres.

REFERENCE VALUES

The determination of a normal range for ECLT is complicated by the non-normal distribution of ECLT values in normal subjects, some individuals displaying values significantly greater than the majority of normal subjects, therefore a reference range is determined by assay of normal plasma samples, followed by log transformation and determination of the geometric mean plus and minus 2 standard deviations from this mean.

CONTROL AND CALIBRATION PROCEDURES

Quality control is not easy to monitor by traditional means as major sources of error are patient selection and preparation as well as in the handling of samples. Quality assurance is maintained by rigid control over all preanalytical variables as well as in the correct performance of the assay. However, quality control may be enhanced by use of control plasmas which are either snap-frozen and stored at − 70 °C, or snap-frozen then freeze-dried and stored at − 20 °C. Ten lyophilized plasmas issued to laboratories participating in ECAT studies showed inter-laboratory coefficients of variation for ECLT ranging from 13.7% to 30.0%.

References

1. Sherry S, Lindemeyer RI, Fletcher AP, Alkjaersig N. Studies on enhanced fibrinolytic activity in man. J Clin Invest 1959; 38: 810–22.
2. Kowalski E, Kopec M, Niewiarowski S. An evaluation of the euglobulin method of determining fibrinolysis. J Clin Pathol 1959; 12: 215–18.
3. Preston FE. Automated clot lysis time. In: Davidson JF, Samama MM, Desnoyers PC, eds. Progress in chemical fibrinolysis and thrombolysis. New York: Raven Press, 1976; vol. II, pp. 24–35.
4. Urano T, Sakakibosa K, Rydzewski A, Urano S, Takada Y, Takada A. Relationship between the euglobulin clot lysis time and the level of tissue plasminogen activator and plasminogen activator inhibitor 1. Thromb Haemostas 1990; 63(1): 82–6.
5. Cooper PC, Preston FE, Greaves M. The relationship of the euglobulin clot lysis time to tissue plasminogen activator and tissue plasminogen activator–inhibitor. Leiden Fibrinolysis Workshop 1986 (abstract).
6. Booth NA, Bennett B, Wijngaards G, Grieve JHK. A new life-long haemorrhagic disorder due to excess plasminogen activator. Blood 1983; 61(2): 267–75.
7. Jorgensen M, Bonnevie-Nielsen V. Increased concentration of the fast-acting plasminogen activator inhibitor in plasma associated with familial venous thrombosis. Br J Haematol 1987; 65: 175–80.
8. Brommer EJP. Delayed fibrinolysis: a cause of thrombosis? Haemostasis 1985; 15: 247–53.
9. Engesser L, Brommer EJP, Kluft C, Briet E. Elevated plasminogen activator–inhibitor (PAI), a cause of thrombophilia? A study of 203 patients with familial or sporadic venous thrombophilia. Thromb Haemostas 1989; 62(2): 673–80.

16
Tissue type plasminogen activator antigen (t-PA Ag)

I. JUHAN-VAGUE and M. C. ALESSI

INTRODUCTION

Physiological role

Tissue type plasminogen activator (t-PA) constitutes an important agent in the fibrinolytic pathway. It is synthesized and released continuously into the blood by endothelial cells and then rapidly cleared by the liver. The secreted form, a single-chain glycoprotein composed of 530 amino acids (70 kD), can be converted by plasmin or kallikrein into a double-chain form with one disulphide bond.

Several domains have been distinguished on the molecule: a finger domain homologous to the type I fingers of fibronectin, an epidermal-growth-factor-like domain, two 'kringle' domains similar to the triple disulphide bound structures found in many plasma proteins, a connecting peptide between the second kringle and the plasmin cleavage site and the carboxyl terminal domain constituting the chain bearing the active site.

The physiological role of t-PA is to activate plasminogen to plasmin which degrades fibrin to soluble degradation products. Fibrinolysis appears to be regulated by specific molecular interactions between t-PA and fibrin as well as between plasmin and α_2-antiplasmin. Because fibrin is required as a cofactor, the activation of plasminogen can occur only on the fibrin surface (for review see ref. 1).

Pathophysiological role

Circulating t-PA levels are thought to have a major effect on fibrinolytic potential, and proper regulation of the t-PA is essential. Decreased release of t-PA has been associated with thrombosis and high t-PA levels with bleeding.

Various tests have been designed to evaluate t-PA release. Different aspects of the response are probably measured depending on the stimulus used, e.g. venostasis[2], desamino-8-D-arginine vasopressin (DDAVP) injection[3] or physical exercise[4]. The capacity of the endothelium to release t-PA can be assessed by comparing either t-PA activity or antigen level before and after stimulation.

Circadian variations in t-PA antigen have been described in relation with variations in plasminogen activator inhibitor 1 (PAI-1). Increase in t-PA antigen concentration has been reported in the elderly and in inflammatory syndrome, in association with several clinical conditions involving increased PAI-1 concentration. The association of hyperfibrinolysis with haemorrhage is usually attributed to a lack of inhibitor, but a tendency to bleeding has also been observed in patients displaying high t-PA release. Venostasis revealed defects in t-PA release in patients with severe von Willebrand disease and abnormally low release of t-PA has been reported in 10–20% of patients with recurrent deep vein thrombosis (for review see ref. 5). The pathological significance of these defects is not well understood.

METHODOLOGY

t-PA activity in whole blood or plasma varies due to reactions between t-PA and inhibitors resulting in formation of t-PA inhibitor complexes. Immunological determination of t-PA allows a total quantification of circulating t-PA.

Efforts to develop assay procedures for t-PA antigen in plasma have been under way for 8 years and several techniques have been described (for specifications and references, see Table 16.1). The earliest methods were radioimmunoassays but they were soon replaced by enzyme-linked immunosorbent assays (ELISA) which have the advantage of using a stable enzyme label. The switch to ELISA was concomitant with improvements in calibrator preparation, in antibody sources and in the buffer as well as the tracer. Current commercially available kits contain stable and reproducible reagents.

Techniques

Radioimmunoassay

Radioimmunoassay based on ^{125}I-labelled antibodies against t-PA (^{125}I-Ab) was the first method to be used. Briefly samples were incubated in polystyrene tubes or microtitre plates coated with IgG from goat or rabbit antiserum. After washing, ^{125}I-Ab was added. Finally, after another wash, radioactivity on the walls of the recipient was counted in a γ-scintillator. Results were evaluated by comparison with a standard curve constructed with pure t-PA.

In one variant of this technique, the sample, antiserum and ^{125}I-t-PA were first incubated. Next anti-IgG immobilized covalently to Sepharose was added and the bound and free fractions were separated by sedimentation through 10% sucrose or centrifugation. Finally radioactivity in the solid phase was counted.

Table 16.1 Characteristics of the assays published

	Holmberg: Scand J Clin Lab Invest 1982, 42: 347	MacGregor: Thromb Res 1983, 31: 461	Rijken: J Lab Clin Med 1983, 101: 274	Matsuo: Analyt Biochem 1983, 135: 58	Bergsdorf: Thromb Haemostas 1983, 50: 740	Urden: Scand J Clin Invest 1984, 44: 495	Rijken: Thromb Res 1984, 33: 145	Holvoet: Thromb Haemostas 1985, 54: 282	Kaizu: Thromb Res 1985, 40: 91	Takada: Thromb Res 1986, 42: 63	Wun: Blood 1987, 69: 1348
Method	RIA	RIA	RIA	RIA	RIA	RIA	EIA	EIA	EIA	EIA	RIA
Antibodies	Goat IgG	Rabbit IgG	Rabbit IgG	Goat IgG	Rabbit IgG	Rabbit IgG	Rabbit IgG, Goat IgG	Monoclonal	Monoclonal	Rabbit F(ab')2 monoclonal	Rabbit IgG
t-PA	Melanoma	Melanoma	Melanoma	Melanoma	Melanoma	Melanoma	Melanoma	Melanoma	Melanoma	Melanoma	Hela cells
Tracer	^{125}I IgG	^{125}I IgG	^{125}I IgG	BD galactosidase	Peroxidase	^{125}I t-PA	Alkaline phosphatase	Peroxidase	Peroxidase	BD galactosidase	^{125}I IgG
Concentration range (μg/L)	1–20	1–40	1–100	0.1–10	0.05–1.2	1–20	1–100	0.10–10	5–100		0–16
Sensitivity (μg/L)	0.7	2	1	0.1	0.1	0.08	1	0.2	1		0.5
Plasma normal values (μg/L)	2.9 ± 2.1	7.1 ± 1.6	6.6 ± 2.9	1.2 ± 0.3	4.0 ± 1.8	4.4 ± 1.3	8.6 ± 1.9	3.4 ± 0.8		6.3 ± 0.3	6.5 ± 0.3
Within-assay coefficient (%)	3–5	4–6			8–11	4–5	14–18	4–5			
Between-assay coefficient (%)	12	11–15			8–11	5–10	25	6.5			
Fold increase after DDAVP or venous occlusion	2–4	2.5–3.5			3	3–4	3	3			

133

ELISA

ELISA techniques rapidly superseded radioimmunoassay because they are so much easier to perform. Specific IgG or the F (ab')2 fragments were coupled on polystyrene wells in which samples were incubated for a few hours. After washing, peroxidase- or β-D-galactosidase-labelled antibodies were added. Specific substrate (orthophenylene diamine methylumbelliferyl β-D galactoside) was then added for various periods of time depending on the assay. The relationship between t-PA and fluorescence intensity or coloration was measured using a spectrofluorometer (ex 360 nm, em 450 nm) or a spectrophotometer (492 nm) respectively.

Rijken et al.[6] described a three-step ELISA procedure with the last step consisting in the use of a rabbit anti-(goat) IgG labelled with alkaline phosphatase. Holvoet et al.[7] proposed a two-site ELISA using a coating phase comprising the IgG fractions of two monoclonal antibodies directed against different exposed epitopes on the t-PA molecule. They also proposed an ELISA for free t-PA using a murine monoclonal antibody directed against the active site of t-PA[8].

Materials

Calibrator t-PA

t-PA is synthesized and secreted at a much higher level by numerous cultured human cell lines than by endothelial cells. t-PA purified from the culture medium of Bowes melanoma cell line has served as a rich source of calibrator t-PA. Several purification processes have been described. t-PA was first purified using immunoaffinity chromatography with antibodies directed against porcine t-PA, chromatography on arginine Sepharose and gel filtration. Then extraction of t-PA was achieved by three chromatographies using zinc chelate Sepharose and concanavalin A Sepharose, followed by filtration on Sephadex G50. More recently t-PA has been purified by immunoaffinity chromatography using monoclonal antibodies directed against human t-PA.

Wun and Capuano[11] obtained calibrator t-PA from Hela cells stimulated with 12-O-tetradecanoyl phorbol 13 acetate by chromatography on *Erythrina latissima* inhibitor Sepharose 4B. The resulting product was a mixture of the single- and double-chain forms. Purification in the presence of aprotinine allowed production of a 90% pure single-chain form (sct-PA). t-PA has been produced by DNA recombinant technology. Concentrations in the purified preparation were determined by protein quantification and amino acid analysis.

Antibodies

All the assays described up to now have made use of specific antibodies raised in goats or rabbits. IgGs were purified by ammonium sulphate precipitation or from protein A Sepharose. Monoclonal antibodies have also been produced in order to obtain stable and reproducible antibodies.

Quality control and reference values

Gaffney[9] analysed data of ELISA for t-PA performed in 13 different laboratories and observed a high degree of variability in results. Discrepancies were greatest when normal plasma was assayed using the international laboratory standard established in 1983. The International Committee for Thrombosis and Hemostasis (fibrinolysis subcommittee) has recommended that plasma with a known level of t-PA be made available to supplement the current t-PA international standard for the measurement of t-PA in plasma. Reference values obtained with the different assays are summarized in Table 16.1. The mean is around 6–7 ng/ml.

Sample collection

Blood samples should be taken after a 20-min rest period. Since t-PA levels are subject to circadian variations, timing should be carefully standardized and subjects should have a normal day/night rhythm. Cooling does not seem to be necessary. Any anticoagulant is suitable but it is advisable to freeze plasma rapidly and conserve it below −30 °C.

Problems

False positives

The presence of an excess of non-immune IgG can reduce the risk of false positives resulting from the presence of antibodies against IgG or rheumatoid factors in the plasma samples.

Calibrator

Potential discrepancies exist between features of Bowes melanoma t-PA and those of endothelial t-PA as the secretory pathways of these cells are different. t-PA secreted by Bowes melanoma cell line consists of two types differing by three amino acid residues. In the same way recombinant t-PA through the homogeneous polypeptide chain could be aberrantly glycosylated. The concentration amount of single-chain t-PA versus double-chain t-PA should be assessed. Caution should be used when comparing various preparations of t-PA.

Crypticity

Two major problems with current immunoassays were poor recovery and lack of parallelism between the dilution curves constructed in plasma and buffer. However, t-PA in serum free cell culture media requires no manipulation for full detection of antigen and addition of EDTA, poly-L-lysine to plasma improves results[10]. Wun and Capuano[11] have shown that the addition of 0.5 mol/L of lysine or arginine and slight acidification of plasma are highly efficient in revealing the plasma t-PA antigen.

This phenomenon has been attributed to the efficiency of the reaction between t-PA antigen in citrated plasma and immobilized t-PA-specific antibodies. The reaction rate can be considerably enhanced by adding EDTA, lysine or acid. It has been speculated that a large portion of the t-PA in citrated plasma is not readily accessible to the antibody. This portion has been termed 'cryptic'.

COMMERCIALLY AVAILABLE KITS

The assay used in ECAT

ECAT assay for t-PA antigen is an ELISA using polyclonal antibodies and peroxidase substrate (Biopool). This assay appears to be particularly reliable as background due to non-specific immunoglobulin, i.e. rheumatoid factors, is eliminated by determining two optical densities: one in the presence of normal goat IgG (N-well) and the other in the presence of goat anti t-PA IgG (A-well). The t-PA signal corresponds to the difference between the N-well and the A-well. In order to enhance recovery and suppress t-PA crypticity, a dilution buffer composed of saline phosphate containing 1 g/L Tween 20 and 5 mmol/L EDTA is used. This composition is as effective as acidification or lysine. The assay allows direct determination of the immunoreactivity of t-PA alone or complexed with purified inhibitors, i.e. PAI-1, PAI-2, α_2-antiplasmin, C1 inhibitor. Consistently accurate results have been obtained by different laboratories, the 'within' and 'between' assay coefficients being 5% and 8% respectively.

Other commercially available kits

Several ELISA kits are available for the t-PA antigen quantification in plasma. Some use F(ab')2 antibody fragments to prevent interference from rheumatoid factors. Others use monoclonal or polyclonal antibodies. Various types of calibrator t-PA are used; it may be obtained from melanoma cells or recombinant technology. Since most of these assays use an adequate buffer, they feature low detection limits and satisfactory reproducibility (Table 16.2).

Table 16.2 Leading manufacturers

Firms	Kit's name
Biopool	Immulyse t-PA
	Tintelize t-PA
Cabru	t-PA assay kit
Kabi	Coaliza t-PA
Imco	t-PA assay kit
Innogenetics	Innotest t-PA
Stago	Asserachrom t-PA
Monozyme	t-PA assay kit

CONCLUSION

Methods for measuring t-PA antigen in plasma have improved in the past few years. Several techniques have been proposed but little comparative data is available. A complete characterization of each is needed to determine reactivity against all the forms of t-PA as well as calibrator t-PA issued from several sources. A better understanding of the different assays should lead to better interlaboratory correlation.

References

1. Bachmann F. Fibrinolysis, In: Verstraete M, Vermylen J, Lijnen R, Arnout J, eds. Thrombosis and haemostasis. Leuven: Leuven University Press, 1987; 227: 265.
2. Robertson B, Pandolfi M, Nilsson IM. Fibrinolytic capacity in healthy volunteers at different ages as studied by standardized venous occlusion of arms and legs. Acta Med Scand 1972; 191: 199.
3. Brommer EJP, Barrett-Bergshoeff MM, Allen RA, Schicht L, Bertina RM, Schalekamp MADH. The use of desmopressin acetate (DDAVP) as a test of the fibrinolytic capacity of patients, analysis of responders and non-responders. Thromb Haemostas 1982; 48: 156.
4. Cash JD. Control mechanism of activator release. In: Davidson JF, Rowan RM, Samama MM, Desnoyers PC, eds. Progress in Chemical Fibrinolysis and Thrombolysis, vol. 3. New York: Raven Press, 1978; 65.
5. Juhan-Vague I, Aillaud MF, Alessi MC. Biological variation in t-PA activity and antigen. In: Kluft C, ed. Tissue-type plasminogen activator (t-PA): physiological and clinical aspects, vol. 2. Boca Raton, FL: CRC Press, 1988; 69.
6. Rijken DC, Juhan-Vague I, DeCock F, Collen D. Measurement of human tissue-type plasminogen activator by a two-site immunoradiometric assay. J Lab Clin Med 1983; 101: 274.
7. Holvoet P, Cleemput H, Collen D. Assay of human tissue type plasminogen activator (t-PA) with an enzyme linked immunosorbent assay (ELISA) based on three murine monoclonal antibodies to t-PA. Thromb Haemostas 1985; 54: 684.
8. Holvoet P, Boes J, Collen D. Measurement of free, one chain tissue-type plasminogen activator in human plasma with an enzyme-linked immunosorbent assay based on an active site specific murine monoclonal antibody. Blood 1987; 69: 284.
9. Gaffney PJ. Specific assays of plasminogen activators and inhibitors. European School of Hematology: Fibrinolysis, 2–6 October 1989.
10. Ranby M, Nguyen G, Scarabin PY, Samama M. Immunoreactivity of tissue plasminogen activator and of its inhibitor complexes. Thromb Haemostas 1989; 61: 409.
11. Wun TC, Capuano A. Immunoradiometric quantitation of tissue plasminogen activator related antigen in human plasma crypticity phenomenon and relationship to plasma fibrinolysis. Blood 1987; 69: 1348.

17
Tissue-type plasminogen activator activity assay

J. H. VERHEIJEN

INTRODUCTION

Measurement of overall blood fibrinolytic activity was introduced many years ago (for a review see ref. 1), but the measurement of specific components involved in fibrinolytic activity became possible only in the last decade or so. The older methods such as dilute blood clot lysis or euglobulin clot lysis measure overall fibrinolytic activity, which is dependent on plasminogen activator level, both tissue-type plasminogen activator (t-PA) and urokinase-type plasminogen activator (u-PA), plasminogen level, the levels of inhibitors of plasminogen activators such as PAI-1 and PAI-2, the levels of plasmin inhibitors such as α_2-antiplasmin and α_2-macroglobulin and the levels of several other compounds, e.g. histidine-rich glycoprotein, fibrinogen and fibrin(ogen) degradation products. Specific assay of t-PA became feasible after the purification of this enzyme and the production of specific antibodies[2,3]. The development of t-PA assays based on synthetic peptide substrates in the early 1980s made t-PA assays available outside the small circle of specialists.

Measurement of t-PA activity in blood or blood-related fractions is difficult since the levels of the enzyme are generally very low, and many other interfering components are present, so suitable assays have to be very sensitive and specific. Different methods were devised to obtain this high sensitivity and specificity. Almost all procedures have solved the sensitivity problem by using a two-stage process involving conversion of plasminogen to plasmin by t-PA followed by measurement of plasmin activity using a plasmin-specific peptide substrate with a chromogenic or fluorogenic leaving group. To increase sensitivity even further, various enhancers were used that in most cases increase the rate of conversion of plasminogen to plasmin by t-PA[4-9]. The specificity is sometimes increased by using specific antibodies to quench t-PA[5,10,11] or to purify and concentrate t-PA from the sample[8,9,12-14]. Other

139

methods employ the specific fibrin binding properties of t-PA for this purpose[7]. Most of these methods have been relatively successful for measurement of t-PA activity in purified systems. Measurement of t-PA in blood or plasma turned out to be more difficult. It was found that these methods generally did not detect any t-PA activity in normal plasma. Only after some stimulus, such as venous occlusion or treatment with DDAVP, could t-PA activity in plasma be found. Recovery experiments of t-PA added to plasma revealed the cause of this observation: the presence of a specific fast-acting inhibitor of t-PA[10,15-18,43], later better characterized and named PAI-1[19,20,42].

The reaction of t-PA with PAI-1 is essentially irreversible and very rapid with a rate constant of about $10^7 \, mol^{-1} \, L \, s^{-1}$. The continuous release, clearance and complex formation of t-PA and PAI-1 leads *in vivo* to steady-state levels of free active t-PA, free active PAI-1 and inactive t-PA·PAI-1 complexes. The complex formation does not stop after blood collection, whereas release and clearance, of course, no longer continue (Figure 17.1). The result is that lower values of t-PA activity are measured than were actually present *in vivo*, in many cases even no detectable t-PA activity is present. In the first t-PA assays described in literature these effects were not fully recognized since PAI-1 was not yet known at that time. The low activities measured were attributed to the presence of plasmin inhibitors interfering with plasmin activity or having some affinity for t-PA[4,5]. Consequently, methods were devised to remove or prevent the action of plasmin inhibitors; these included euglobulin fractionation and plasma acidification. Later acidification turned out to be a very efficient method to slow down the interaction between PAI-1 and t-PA and acidification of the blood was performed just after collection[22]. Using euglobulin fractionation or plasmin/blood acidification t-PA activity could be detected under normal unstimulated conditions. Activities measured after acidification are much higher than after euglobulin fractionation (Table 17.2) and acidification appears to be the best way to preserve t-PA activity in blood. The currently used methods for t-PA activity assay consists of several steps: first a blood collection and treatment procedure, to minimize *in vitro* effects on t-PA activity; second, an optional concentration procedure often also increasing the specificity; finally the actual assay.

The blood collection procedure is more or less independent of the other steps but of utmost importance (see above) and therefore will be treated in detail later in this chapter.

Several concentration procedures have been described in literature, most often coupled to a particular assay, but some of the general principles are assay-independent and could also be employed in other assay methods. The affinity of t-PA for lysine-Sepharose[6] or immobilized fibrin[7] has been used to purify and concentrate t-PA from plasmin. Several assays use immobilized t-PA-specific antibodies in assays according to the elegant BIA principle[9,12,13]. The actual assays are very similar and involve the conversion of plasminogen to plasmin coupled to the hydrolysis of a plasmin substrate, often in the presence of a stimulating substance. Different chromogenic plasmin substrates are used and several stimulators are used such as soluble fibrin[14,23]. CNBr-digested fibrinogen[5] poly-lysine derivatives[9,24] or coated fibrin[7].

Table 17.1 Assay methods for t-PA in blood

Reference	Blood treatment	Stimulator	Substrate	Remarks
1. Verheijen et al.[5,21]	euglobulin	CNBr digested fbg	S2251	absorption to lysine–Sepharose
2. Wiman et al.[4]	acidified plasma	soluble fibrin	S2251	further development of 1
3. Gyzander et al.[6]	plasma	poly-lysine	S2251	BIA immobilized anti t-PA
4. Verheijen et al.[10]	euglobulin	CNBr digested fbg	S2251	further development of 2
5. Mahmoud et al.[12]	plasma/euglobulin	–	S2390	SOFIA, immobilized fibrin
6. Chmielewska and Wiman[22]	acidified blood	soluble fibrin	S2251	immobilized anti t-PA combined with ELISA
7. Angles-Cano[7]	plasma	fibrin	S2251	immobilized anti t-PA
8. Wojta et al.[14]	plasma	CNBr digested fbg	S2251	combination of 1 and 2
9. Dahl et al.[8]	plasma	polylysine	PL-1	development of 3
10. Nilsson et al.[36]	acidified blood	CNBr digested fbg	S2251	immobilized anti t-PA
11. Eriksson and Risberg[37]	acidified plasma	polylysine	S2251	BIA development of 5
12. Petersen et al.[9]	acidified plasma	TNB-polylysine	S2251	adaptation from 1
13. Mahmoud-Alexandroni et al.[13]	plasma	–	S2251	
14. Chandler et al.[38]	acidified blood	CNBr digested fbg	S2390, spectrozyme PL	
15. Rånby[33]	acidified blood	soluble fibrin	H-D-ButCHT Lys pNA	adaptation from 2, 6
16. Wejkum[34]	two-step acidification	CNBr digested fbg	S2251	adaptation from 1, 2, 10

S2251: H-D-Val-Leu-Lys-pNA
PL-1: H-D-Nleu-CHA-Lys-pNA
Spectrozyme PL: H-D-Nleu-HHT-Lys-pNA
S2390: H-D-Val-Phe-Lys-pNA

141

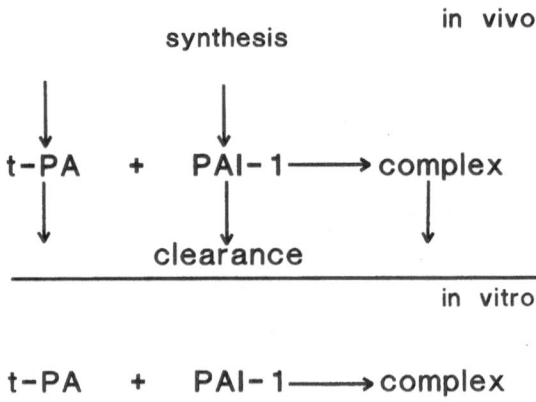

Figure 17.1 Fate of t-PA and PAI-1 *in vivo* and *in vitro*

When the plasmin formation and synthetic substrate hydrolysis are performed simultaneously, this leads to parabolic kinetics[25], meaning that the product formation is linear with the square of the incubation duration (Figure 17.2).

BLOOD COLLECTION AND SAMPLE PREPARATION

The t-PA activity in blood can change very rapidly as a response to physical exercise[26], stress, smoking[27], alcohol[28] and caffeine[29]. Furthermore, the t-PA

Table 17.2 Comparison of plasma values of t-PA activity

Assay method	Blood treatment	Activity (i.u./ml)	Reference
1	euglobulin	0.08	Kluft et al.[29]
2	acidified plasma	0.14	Grant and Lottenberg[39]
1	acidified plasma	1.0	Kohler and Miyashita[40]
1	euglobulin	0.054	Kohler and Miyashita[40]
2	acidified plasma	1.80	Krishnamurti et al.[41]
1	acidified blood	1.59	Chandler et al.[38]
2	acidified plasma	0.11	Wiman et al.[4]
1	euglobulin	0.02	Verheijen et al.[10]; Verheijen[1,11]
6	acidified blood	0.47	Rånby et al.[33]
1, 6	acidified blood	0.39	Nilsson et al.[36]
1, 6	acidified plasma	0.23	Nilsson et al.[36]
8	plasma	<0.2	Wojta et al.[14]
9	plasma	nd	Dahl et al.[8]
5	plasma	nd	Mahmoud et al.[12]
13	plasma	0.01–0.06	Mahmoud-Alexandroni et al.[13]
12	acidified plasma	0–1.05	Petersen et al.[9]
3	plasma	0.16	Gyzander et al.[6]

The assay methods refer to Table 17.1. Activities are expressed in i.u. of t-PA; in some cases this activity had to be calculated from the cited reference using the specific activity of purified t-PA cited in the reference, or of 5×10^5 i.u./mg, when not cited, and a molecular weight of 70 000

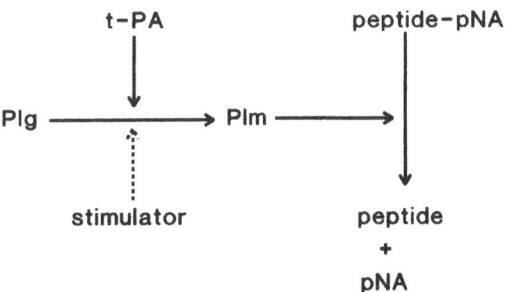

$$[pNA]=k.[t-PA].t^2$$

Figure 17.2 Principle of parabolic rate assay

level is not constant but varies during the day in a 24 h rhythm[30]. In devising studies[31] involving t-PA measurements in groups of patients or controls the above-mentioned complications should be recognized and, if possible, eliminated by standardization.

To prevent the *in vitro* reaction between t-PA and PAI-1, acidification is probably the most attractive option. Early procedures, where blood was acidified to pH 4, gave problems with haemolysis, therefore a two-step procedure has been introduced[32-34]. In the first step the pH is decreased to 6, at which pH the reaction between t-PA and PAI-1 is dramatically decreased but no haemolysis occurs. Plasma is prepared and t-PA is further stabilized by a second addition of acid to a final pH of 3. When plasma is prepared in this way and stored at −70 °C, t-PA activity is stable for months. A detailed description of blood collection and plasma preparation for t-PA activity assays can be found in Kluft and Verheijen[35].

A major disadvantage of this procedure is that blood collected for other purposes cannot be used for t-PA assays. When blood collection cannot be performed as indicated, but information of t-PA activity is still required, it is possible to use acidified plasma instead. This will give lower values for t-PA activity which are very much dependent on rapidity of blood collection and plasma preparation, so standardized procedures are very important. The use of euglobulin fractionation is no longer recommended.

ASSAY METHODS FOR t-PA

Currently employed assay methods for t-PA activity in blood are summarized in Table 17.1. All methods are based on the same principle, the parabolic rate assay as originally described by Drapier *et al.*[25]. The main differences between the methods are the use of different plasmin substrates, rate-enhancers and methods for increasing sensitivity and specificity. Although the original methods often included a particular blood collection and treatment procedure, this was not considered to be an essential part of the method. The method of choice, two-step acidification, can probably be combined with many, if not all, assays.

A rigorous comparison of the results obtained by different methods has not yet been performed, but some data are available and can be found in Table 17.2. In order to compare data they were all converted to i.u. of t-PA using a specific activity of 5×10^5 i.u./mg and a molecular weight of 7×10^4 for t-PA.

As can be seen from this table, activities found in euglobulin fractions are much lower than in acid-treated blood or plasma. Even in acid-treated blood or plasma a wide range of t-PA activities has been found, most probably representing differences in treatment of subjects and time of sampling. Results of assays should be expressed as international units of t-PA referring to the standard used. The use of an established reference preparation rather than manufacturers' standards is recommended when using kits. Upon publication always specify how blood was collected, how plasma was prepared (see ref. 35) and which standard was used.

MATERIALS NEEDED FOR t-PA ASSAY

Several companies sell either separate reagents of use or kits containing all necessary components (see Chapter 27). The quality of the plasminogen is important; it should not contain much plasmin activity, leading to high blanks and a higher detection limit.

COMMENTS

During the ECAT studies, for determination of the t-PA activity plasma was prepared as usual, followed by euglobulin fractionation. t-PA activity was measured in the euglobulin fraction using the method of Verheijen[5]. Although the results were found to be valuable, it appeared that standardizing the assay was difficult. The main problem is most likely the *in vitro* reaction between t-PA and inhibitors which occurs during the handling of blood and plasma before the euglobulin fractionation.

Therefore, we recommend acidification of blood and plasma (Table 17.3) which largely prevents the *in vitro* inhibition and improves standardization.

Table 17.3

Blood + acidified citrate 9 + 1 (final pH ≈ 6)
Plasma preparation
Plasma + 1 mol/L HCl 15 + 1 (final pH ≈ 3)
Store at −70 °C
Thaw at 37 °C for 5 min (or fixed time period identical for all samples)
Place in crushed ice/water mixture until use

For details see ref. 35

It has become evident in recent years that measurement of only t-PA activity is probably of limited use. Its value is a result of the levels of at least t-PA and PAI-1. Combination of both assays is recommended (see also t-PA antigen and PAI assays).

References

1. Verheijen JH. Purification, assay and standardization of t-PA. In: Kluft C, ed. Tissue-type plasminogen activator (t-PA): physiological and clinical aspects, vol. 1. Boca Raton, FL: CRC Press, 1988; 123–44.
2. Rijken DC, Wijngaards G, Zaal-De Jong M, Welbergen J. Purification and partial characterization of plasminogen activator from human uterine tissue. Biochim Biophys Acta 1979; 580: 140–53.
3. Rijken DC, Wijngaards G, Welbergen J. Relationship between tissue plasminogen activator and the activators in blood and vascular wall. Thromb Res 1980; 18: 815–30.
4. Wiman B, Mellbring G, Rånby M. Plasminogen activator release during venous stasis and exercise as determined by a new specific assay. Clin Chem Acta 1983; 127: 279–88.
5. Verheijen JH, Mullaart E, Chang GTG, Kluft C, Wijngaards G. A simple, sensitive spectrophotometric assay for extrinsic (tissue-type) plasminogen activator applicable to measurements in plasma. Thromb Haemostas 1982; 48: 266–9.
6. Gyzander E, Eriksson E, Teger-Nilsson AC. A sensitive assay for tissue plasminogen activator activity in plasma using adsorption on lysine sepharose. Thromb Res 1984; 35: 547–58.
7. Angles-Cano E. A spectrophotometric solid phase fibrin tissue plasminogen activator activity assay: sofia-t-PA for high fibrin affinity tissue plasminogen activators. Anal Biochem 1986; 153: 201–10.
8. Dahl KH, Holst J, Smith P, Gogstad GO. Functional measurement of t-PA in plasma using a bead immuno chromogenic assay (BICA). Fibrinolysis 1987; 1: 83–9.
9. Petersen LC, Handest P, Brender J, Selmer J, Jorgensen M, Thorsen S. A sensitive solid-phase immunosorbent assay for tissue-type plasminogen activator activity in plasma using trinitrobenzoylated poly-D-lysine as a stimulator for plasminogen activation. Thromb Haemostas 1987; 57: 205–11.
10. Verheijen JH, Chang GTG, Kluft C. Evidence for the occurrence of a fast-acting inhibitor for tissue-type plasminogen activator in human plasma. Thromb Haemostas 1984; 51: 392–5.
11. Verheijen JH. Tissue plasminogen activator and fast-acting plasminogen activator inhibitor in plasma. In: DiSaboto G, ed. Methods in enzymology, vol. 163. San Diego, CA: Academic Press, 1988; 302–9.
12. Mahmoud M, Gaffney PJ. Bioimmunoassay (BIA) of tissue plasminogen activator t-PA and its specific inhibitor t-PA/INH. Thromb Haemostas 1985; 53: 356–9.
13. Mahmoud-Alexandroni M, Heath AB, Gaffney PJ. Sensitive and direct assays for functionally active plasminogen activators (tissue-type and urokinase-type) in plasma. Am J Clin Pathol 1989; 92: 308–14.
14. Wojta J, Turcu L, Wagner OF, Korninger C, Binder BR. Evaluation of fibrinolytic capacity by a combined assay system for tissue-type plasminogen activator antigen and function using monoclonal anti-tissue-plasminogen activator antibodies. J Lab Clin Med 1987; 109: 665–71.
15. Kruithof EKO, Ransjin A, Bachmann F. Inhibition of tissue plasminogen activator by human plasma. Prog. Fibrinolysis 1983; 6: 365–9.
16. Chmielewska, J. Rånby M, Wiman B. Evidence for a rapid inhibitor to tissue plasminogen activator in plasma. Thromb Res 1983; 31: 427–36.
17. Juan-Vague I, Moerman B, De Cock F, Aillaud MF, Collen D. Plasma levels of a specific inhibitor of tissue type plasminogen activator and urokinase in normal and pathological conditions. Thromb Res 1984; 33: 523–30.
18. Thorsen S, Philips M. Isolation of tissue-type plasminogen activator inhibitor complexes from human plasma: evidence for a rapid plasminogen activator inhibitor. Biochim Biophys Acta 1984; 802: 111–18.
19. Kruithof EKO. Plasminogen activator inhibitors. A review. Enzyme 1988; 40: 113–21.

20. Sprengers ED, Kluft C. Plasminogen activator inhibitors. Blood 1987; 69: 381–7.
21. Verheijen JH, Nieuwenhuizen W, Wijngaards G. Activation of plasminogen by tissue activator is increased specifically in the presence of certain soluble fibrin(ogen) fragments. Thromb Res 1982b; 27: 377–85.
22. Chmielewska J, Wiman B: Determination of tissue plasminogen activator and its fast inhibitor in plasma. Clin Chem 1986; 32: 482–5.
23. Rånby M, Norrman B, Wallén P. A sensitive assay for tissue plasminogen activator. Thromb Res 1982; 27: 743–9.
24. Allen RA. An enhancing effect of polylysine on the activation of plasminogen. Thromb Haemostas 1982; 47: 41–5.
25. Drapier JC, Tenu JP, Lemaire G, Petit JF. Regulation of plasminogen activator secretion in mouse peritoneal macrophages. I. Role of serum studied by a new spectrophotometric assay for plasminogen activators. Biochimie 1979; 61: 463–71.
26. Vene N, Stegnar M. Tissue-type plasminogen activator and plasminogen activator inhibitor-1 after exercise — comparison to venous occlusion and DDAVP. Fibrinolysis 1990; 4: 105–7.
27. Allen RA, Kluft C, Brommer EJP. Acute effect of smoking on fibrinolysis: increase in the activity level of circulating extrinsic tissue-type plasminogen activator. Eur J Clin Invest 1984; 14: 354–61.
28. Veenstra J, Te Wierik E, Kluft C. Alcohol and fibrinolysis. Fibrinolysis 1990; 4: 64–8.
29. Kluft C, Kooistra T, Veenstra J, Schaafsma G. Effects of coffee and caffeine on tissue-type plasminogen activator and its fast-acting inhibitor, PAI-1, *in vivo* and *in vitro*. Fibrinolysis 1990; 4: 74–5.
30. Kluft C, Jie AFH, Rijken DC, Verheijen JH. Daytime fluctuations in blood of tissue type plasminogen activator (t-PA) and its fast acting inhibitor (PAI-1). Thromb Haemostas 1988; 59: 329–32.
31. Peternel P, Stegnar M, Salobir U, Salobir B, Keber D, Vene N. Shift work and circadian rhythm of blood fibrinolytic parameters. Fibrinolysis 1990; 4: 113–15.
32. De Maat MPM, Kluft C, De Boer K, Knot EAR, Jie AFH. Acid treatment of plasma for the inactivation of plasminogen activator inhibitor-1 (PAI-1). Thromb Res 1988; 52: 425–30.
33. Rånby N, Sundell IB, Nilsson TK. Blood collection in strong acidic citrate anticoagulant used in a study of dietary influence on basal t-PA activity. Thromb Haemostas 1989; 62: 917–22.
34. Wejkum, L, Rosen S, Sorskog L, Brandt B, Chmielewska J. Blood sampling and determination of tissue plasminogen activator activity with CoA-set t-PA. Fibrinolysis 1990; 4: 152–4.
35. Kluft C, Verheijen JH. Leiden Fibrinolysis Working Party: blood collection and handling procedures for assessment of tissue-type plasminogen activator (t-PA) and plasminogen activator inhibitor-1 (PAI-1). Fibrinolysis 1990; 4: 155–61.
36. Nilsson K, Rosen S, Friberger P. A new kit for the determination of tissue plasminogen activator and its inhibitor in blood. Fibrinolysis 1987; 1: 163–8.
37. Eriksson E, Risberg B. Measurement of tissue plasminogen activator in plasma. A comparison of three methods and description of a new improved technique. Thromb Res 1987; 46: 213–23.
38. Chandler WL, Schmer G, Stratton JR. Optimum conditions for the stabilization and measurement of tissue plasminogen activator activity in human plasma. J Lab Clin Med 1989; 113: 362–71.
39. Grant MB, Lottenberg R. Desmopressin stimulates parallel norepinephrine and tissue-type plasminogen activator release in normal subjects and patients with diabetes mellitus. Thromb Haemostas 1988; 59: 269–72.
40. Kohler M, Miyashita C. Problems in determining parameters of the fibrinolytic system: circadian variations of tissue type plasminogen activator and plasminogen activator inhibitor. Klin Wochenschr 1988; 66: 62–7.
41. Krishnamurti C, Tang DB, Barr CF, Alving BM. Plasminogen activator and plasminogen activator inhibitor activities in a reference population. Am J Clin Pathol 1988; 89: 747–52.
42. Kruithof EKO. Plasminogen activator inhibitor type 1: biochemical, biological and clinical aspects. Fibrinolysis 1988; 2: 59–70.
43. Kruithof EKO, Tran-Thang C, Ransijn A, Bachmann F. Demonstration of a fast acting inhibitor of plasminogen activators in human plasma. Blood 1984; 64: 907–13.

18
Plasminogen activator inhibitor activity assay

E. K. O. KRUITHOF

INTRODUCTION

Plasminogen activator inhibitor type 1 (PAI-1) is one of the principal inhibitors of the fibrinolytic enzyme system. It is a very efficient inhibitor of tissue-type plasminogen activator (t-PA) and urokinase (u-PA), with second-order rate constants ($> 10^7 \, \text{mol}^{-1} \, \text{s}^{-1}$) among the fastest described for protease-inhibitor reactions. High plasma levels of this inhibitor are associated with a poor prognosis in patients with septicaemia and in survivors of myocardial infarction, and with postoperative thrombosis in patients with elective hip surgery. Several recent reviews give an overview of the clinical aspects and the biochemistry and molecular and cellular biology of PAI-1[1-7].

Many different activity assays have been developed for PAI-1. Most are based upon the inhibition of exogenously added PA. Endogenous t-PA also reacts with PAI-1, and PAI activity assays only reflect the difference in PAI-1 and t-PA levels. In morning samples the effect of endogenous t-PA is relatively small, but after exercise or venous stasis endogenous t-PA may even exceed PAI-1. The amount of added PA is of paramount importance and should exceed that of PAI. However, to enable a precise assessment of the difference between added and recovered PA activity, the excess should not be too large.

The incubation time should be chosen long enough to enable an almost complete reaction of PA with PAI-1, and short enough that the contribution of other plasma protease inhibitors such as α_2-antiplasmin, α_1-protease inhibitor, C'1-inhibitor and α_2-macroglobulin is negligible. Incubation times between 5 and 10 min in undiluted plasma offer a suitable compromise. Termination of the inhibition reaction has been achieved by euglobulin precipitation of t-PA[8], fibrin adsorption of t-PA[9], sample dilution[10,11] or acidification and dilution[12]. Residual activity has been measured on fibrin

147

plates or by chromogenic substrate assays. Titration assays using different concentrations of added PA may offer more reliable results, but are time-consuming. For that reason most assays use one PA concentration and dilute the sample when PAI activity is too high.

An alternative approach to measuring PAI activity is to add an excess of t-PA or urokinase (u-PA) to human plasma and to quantify the increase in concentration of PA/PAI complexes[13-15].

Depending on the PA used, PAI activity is expressed in t-PA inhibitory units or u-PA inhibitory units. As one u-PA inhibitory unit is roughly equivalent to eight t-PA inhibitory units the species of PA used should be clearly stated.

It has to be stressed that most PAI activity assays are well suited to measure elevated PAI activities in plasma, but are unsuited to detect PAI deficiencies (e.g. in patients with haemorrhagic syndromes, ref. 16).

METHOD OF ASSAY

Principles and assay characteristics

Most PAI activity assays employed to date correspond to the following general description: One volume of t-PA (40 U/ml) is incubated for 15 min at room temperature with one volume of plasma and then acidified and diluted to destroy antiplasmin activity and block further inhibition of t-PA. Residual t-PA activity is measured in microtitre plates by an indirect chromogenic substrate assay (for more details see Chapter 17). Samples containing more than approximately 30 U/ml should be diluted (preferably with PAI depleted plasma). Table 18.1 summarizes the different PAI activity assays that have been developed. A systematic comparison of the different assays has not yet been made, but in one recent comparative study Alessi et al.[17] obtained a good correlation between a t-PA-based titration assay, a commercial t-PA-based one-point assay and a u-PA-based one-point assay. The slope of the different assays, however, was significantly different. Table 18.2 gives a list of commercial suppliers of PAI activity assays.

Blood collection

Blood should be collected from resting (20 min) subjects by clean venipuncture. In view of the strong diurnal variation of PAI activity the blood collection time should be standardized. Blood can be collected in standard plastic or siliconized tubes containing 0.1 volume of 0.1 mol/L sodium citrate, pH 4.5 (other anticoagulant mixtures may also be suitable). The tubes are immediately placed on ice and centrifuged (20 min, 2000 g, 4 °C) as soon as possible. Immediately thereafter the middle layer of the plasma is collected and snap-frozen in aliquots and stored at −70 °C. A detailed description of suitable blood collection procedures is given by Kluft and Verheijen[18]. (See also Chapter 2.)

Table 18.1 Assay methods for PAI activity in human plasma

Reference	PA used	Assay type
Chmielewska and Wiman[11]	t-PA	indirect chromogenic substrate
Eriksson et al.[12]	t-PA	indirect chromogenic substrate
Juhan-Vague et al.[8]	t-PA	fibrin plate
Jørgensen and Bonnevie-Nielsen[13]	t-PA	Complex formation, SDS-PAGE
Korninger et al.[20]	t-PA	indirect chromogenic substrate
Kruithof et al.[9]	t-PA	fibrin plate
Mahmoud and Gaffney[21]	t-PA	immune adsorption, indirect chromogenic substrate
Masson and Anglés-Cano[22]	t-PA	fibrin adsorption, indirect chromogenic substrate
Nilsson et al.[23]	t-PA	indirect chromogenic substrate
Rydzewski et al.[14]	t-PA	complex formation, ELISA
Schleef et al.[15]	t-PA	complex formation, IRMA
Speiser et al.[24]	t-PA	indirect chromogenic substrate
Stief et al.[25]	u-PA	indirect chromogenic substrate
Verheijen et al.[10]	t-PA	indirect chromogenic substrate

Table 18.2 Companies selling products of use for PAI activity assays

American Diagnostics	Diagnostica Stago
Behringwerke	Kabi Vitrum Diagnostica
Biopool	

Normal values

The distribution of PAI activity values in a control group is skewed and can be normalized by logarithmic conversion[11,17,19]. PAI activity values depend on the assay type and the PA used, are different between men and women, increase with age and correlate with body mass index. Laboratories must establish their own normal range for the particular assay method while taking into consideration the details (age, sex) of patients under investigation. Furthermore as PAI activity shows a strong diurnal variation, the blood collection time should be standardized.

References

1. Sprengers ED, Kluft C. Plasminogen activator inhibitors. Blood 1987; 69: 381–7.
2. Loskutoff DJ, Sawdey M, Mimuro J. Type 1 plasminogen activator inhibitor. Progr Hemostas Thromb 1988; 9: 87–115.
3. Kruithof EKO. Plasminogen activator inhibitor 1: biochemical, biological and clinical aspects. Fibrinolysis 1988; 2 suppl. 2: 59–70.
4. Kruithof EKO. Plasminogen activator inhibitor 1 and its relation to thrombosis. Med Razgl 1990; 29 suppl. 1: 43–52.
5. Saksela O, Rifkin DB. Cell associated plasminogen activation: regulation and physiological functions. Ann Rev Cell Biol 1988; 4: 93–126.
6. Andreasen PA, Georg B, Lund LR, Riccio A, Stacey SN. Plasminogen activator inhibitors, hormonally regulated serpins. Mol Cell Endocrinol 1990; 68: 1–19.
7. Leiden Fibrinolysis Workshop 3 on life style and fibrinolysis. Fibrinolysis 1990; 4 suppl. 2: 47–161.

8. Juhan-Vague I, Moerman B, De Cock F, Aillaud MF, Collen D. Plasma levels of a specific inhibitor of tissue-type plasminogen activator (and urokinase) in normal and pathological conditions. Thromb Res 1984; 33: 523–30.
9. Kruithof EKO, Tran-Thang C, Ransijn A, Bachmann F. Demonstration of a fast-acting inhibitor of plasminogen activators in human plasma. Blood 1984; 64: 907–13.
10. Verheijen JH, Chang GTG, Kluft C. Evidence for the occurrence of a fast-acting inhibitor for tissue-type plasminogen activator in human plasma. Thromb Haemostas 1984; 51: 392–5.
11. Chmielewska J, Wiman B. Determination of tissue plasminogen activator and its 'fast' inhibitor in plasma. Clin Chem 1986; 32: 482–5.
12. Eriksson E, Rånby M, Gyzander E, Risberg B. Determination of plasminogen activator inhibitor in plasma using t-PA and a chromogenic single-point poly-D-lysine stimulated assay. Thromb Res 1988; 50: 91–101.
13. Jørgensen M, Bonnevie-Nielsen V. Increased concentration of the fast-acting plasminogen activator inhibitor in plasma associated with familial venous thrombosis. Br J Haematol 1987; 65: 175–80.
14. Rydzewski A, Takada Y, Takada A. Determination of plasminogen activator inhibitor-1 (PAI-1) in plasma using two different anticoagulants and methods. Thromb Res 1989; 55: 285–9.
15. Schleef RR, Sinha M, Loskutoff D J. Immunoradiometric assay to measure the binding of a specific inhibitor to tissue-type plasminogen activator. J Lab Clin Med 1985; 106: 408–15.
16. Diéval J, Nguyen G, Gross S, Delobel J, Kruithof EKO. A lifelong bleeding disorder associated with a deficiency of plasminogen activator inhibitor type 1. Blood 1991; 77: 528–32.
17. Alessi MC, Gaussem P, Juhan-Vague I, Aiach M, Musitelli JJ, Lenz P, Keuper H. The determination of functional plasminogen activator inhibitors based on the inhibition of urokinase: PAI normal range and circadian variations in healthy donors; comparison with other methods. Fibrinolysis 1990; 4: 177–81.
18. Kluft C, Verheijen JH. Leiden fibrinolysis working party: Blood collection and handling procedures for the assessment of tissue-type plasminogen activator and plasminogen activator inhibitor 1. Fibrinolysis 1990; 4 suppl. 2: 155–61.
19. Kruithof EKO, Gudinchet A, Bachmann F. Plasminogen activator inhibitor 1 and plasminogen activator inhibitor 2 in various disease states. Thromb Haemostas 1988; 59: 7–12.
20. Korninger C, Wagner O, Binder BR. Tissue plasminogen activator inhibitor in human plasma: development of a functional assay system and demonstration of a correlating $M_r = 50\,000$ antiactivator. J Lab Clin Med 1985; 105: 718–24.
21. Mahmoud M, Gaffney PJ. Bioimmunoassay of tissue plasminogen activator and its specific inhibitor. Thromb Haemostas 1985; 53: 356–9.
22. Masson C, Anglés-Cano E. Quantification de l'inhibiteur spécifique (PAI-1) de l'activateur tissulaire du plasminogène (t-PA) dans le plasma. Ann Biol Clin 1989; 47: 269–74.
23. Nilsson IM, Ljungnér H, Tengborn L. Two different mechanisms in patients with venous thrombosis and defective fibrinolysis: low concentration of plasminogen activator or increased concentration of plasminogen activator inhibitor. Br Med J 1985; 290: 1453–6.
24. Speiser W, Bowry S, Anders E, Binder BR, Müller-Berghaus G. Method for the determination of the fast-acting plasminogen activator inhibitor capacity in plasma, platelets and endothelial cells. Thromb Res 1986; 44: 503–15.
25. Stief TW, Lenz P, Becker U, Heimburger N. Determination of plasminogen activator inhibitor capacity of human plasma in presence of oxidants: a novel principle. Thromb Res 1988; 50: 559–73.

19
Plasminogen activator inhibitor antigen

E. K. O. KRUITHOF

INTRODUCTION

Plasminogen activator inhibitor type 1 (PAI-1) antigen assays are not as widely used as PAI activity assays (see Chapter 18) and clinical experience with these assays is limited. The presence in plasma of several distinct forms of PAI-1, and the fact that the PAI-1 antigen assays developed to date measure these forms with different efficacy, render interpretation and comparison of PAI-1 antigen data more complicated. Four distinct forms of PAI-1 have been identified: active, latent, t-PA- or u-PA-bound and proteolytically degraded. For PAI-1 antigen measurements in human plasma the active, latent and t-PA-bound forms are the most important ones. Conformational changes in the PAI-1 molecule upon conversion from active to latent[1] or upon reaction with PAs are considerable and many monoclonal antibodies preferentially recognize one form of PAI-1. As a consequence the results of PAI antigen assay are critically dependent on the assay being used (Table 19.1). In human blood two distinct compartments for PAI-1 have been identified: plasma and platelets. In healthy individuals the amount of PAI-1 antigen in platelets is approximately ten-fold higher than in plasma. However, as platelet PAI-1 is only 5–10% active, and plasma PAI-1 50–80%, the contribution of platelets to total PAI-1 activity in blood is only approximately 60%[2]. To specifically measure plasma PAI-1 antigen, the contribution of platelets should be kept as low as possible. This can be achieved by collecting plasma on anticoagulant/antiaggregant mixtures[3] or by careful treatment of the plasma after blood collection.

Table 19.1 Specificity of assay methods for PAI antigen in human plasma

Reference	Assay type	Specificity
Biopool Immulyse[6]	ELISA	active = latent > t-PA bound
Biopool Tintelize[6]	ELISA	active = t-PA bound > latent
Booth et al.[7]	ELISA	active = latent
De Clerck et al.[2]	ELISA	active = latent > t-PA-bound
De Clerck et al.[8]	ELISA	only t-PA-bound
	ELISA	active = t-PA-bound
Kruithof et al.[9]	RIA	active = latent = t-PA-bound
Monozyme PAI-1[6]	ELISA	latent > t-PA-bound > active
Urdén et al.[10]	RIA	active = latent = t-PA-bound

METHOD OF ASSAY

Principle and assay characteristics

Two types of PAI antigen assays have been described: radioimmunoassays (RIA) and enzyme-linked immunosorbent assays (ELISA). Several antigenically distinct forms of PAI-1 exist and the results of antigen assays using monoclonal antibodies are strongly dependent on the specific antibody used. The specificity of the published assays is given in Table 19.1. ELISAs are easier to accommodate in routine laboratory practice and are to be preferred over the RIAs. The specificity of the assay is quite important for the end-result. For the measurement of PAI-1 antigen in plasma, ideally one would want to have an assay that either is specific for active PAI-1 or measures all forms of PAI-1 with equal sensitivity. At present such assays are not available. Assays that preferentially measure active PAI-1 are less sensitive to contamination by platelet PAI-1, but do not offer more information than PAI activity assays. Total PAI-1 antigen measurements may better discriminate between patient groups and normals, but require special care during blood collection. The choice of the particular PAI-1 antigen assay thus depends on the aims of the project under study.

Table 19.2 gives a list of commercial suppliers of PAI antigen assays.

Blood collection

Blood should be collected from resting (20 min) subjects by clean venipuncture. In view of the strong diurnal variation of PAI antigen the blood collection time should be standardized. As platelets contain a large excess of PAI-1 over plasma, care should be taken to limit platelet release reactions as much as possible. Rapid cooling of the blood prior to centrifugation is critical. The

Table 19.2 Companies selling PAI antigen assay kits

American Diagnostic	Biopool
Monozyme	Kabi Diagnostica

use of platelet stabilization procedures (e.g. see Chapter 3) may further reduce the platelet contribution to measured PAI-1 antigen levels. Blood can be collected in standard plastic or siliconized tubes containing 0.1 volume of 0.1 mol/L sodium citrate, pH 4.5 (other anticoagulant mixtures may also be suitable), immediately placed on ice and centrifuged (20 min, 2000 g, 4 °C) as soon as possible. Immediately thereafter the middle layer of the plasma is collected and snap-frozen in aliquots and stored at −70 °C. A detailed description of suitable blood collection procedures is given by Kluft and Verheijen[4].

Normal values

The distribution of PAI antigen values in a control group is skewed and can be normalized by logarithmic conversion[5]. PAI antigen values depend critically upon the assay (which should be given with the results) and upon the PAI-1 standard preparation used. No international PAI-1 antigen standard is available yet. Some studies observed that PAI antigen levels are different between men and women, increase with age and correlate with body mass index. In view of these results laboratories must establish their own normal range for the particular assay method while taking into consideration the characteristics (age, sex) of the patients under investigation. Furthermore as PAI-1 antigen levels show a strong diurnal variation, the blood collection time should be standardized.

References

1. Hekman CM, Loskutoff DJ. Endothelial cells produce a latent inhibitor of plasminogen activators that can be activated by denaturants. J Biol Chem 1985; 260: 11581–7.
2. De Clerck PJ, Alessi MC, Verstreken M, Kruithof EKO, Juhan-Vague I, Collen D. Measurement of plasminogen activator inhibitor 1 in biologic fluids with a murine monoclonal antibody-based enzyme-linked immunosorbent assay. Blood 1988; 71: 220–5.
3. Juhan-Vague I, Alessi MC, Fossat C, De Clerck PJ, Kruithof EKO. Plasma determination of plasminogen activator inhibitor 1 antigen must be performed in blood collected on antiplatelet/anticoagulant mixture. Thromb Haemostas 1987; 58: 1096.
4. Kluft C, Verheijen JH. Leiden fibrinolysis working party: Blood collection and handling procedures for the assessment of tissue-type plasminogen activator and plasminogen activator inhibitor 1. Fibrinolysis 1990; 4 suppl. 2: 155–61.
5. Kruithof EKO, Gudinchet A, Bachmann F. Plasminogen activator inhibitor 1 and plasminogen activator inhibitor 2 in various disease states. Thromb Haemostas 1988; 59: 7–12.
6. Kluft C, Jie AFH. Comparison of specificities of antigen assays for plasminogen activator inhibitor 1. Fibrinolysis 1990; 4 suppl. 2: 136–7.
7. Booth NA, Simpson AJ, Croll A, Bennett B, McGregor IR. Plasminogen activator inhibitor (PAI-1) in plasma and platelets. Br J Haematol 1988; 70: 327–33.
8. De Clerck PJ, Verstreken M, Collen D. Measurement of different forms of plasminogen activator inhibitor 1 using various monoclonal antibody-based enzyme-linked immunosorbent assays. Fibrinolysis 1990; 4 suppl. 2: 132–3.
9. Kruithof EKO, Nicoloso G, Bachmann F. Plasminogen activator inhibitor 1: development of a radioimmunoassay and observations on its plasma concentration during venous occlusion and after platelet aggregation. Blood 1987; 70: 1645–53.
10. Urdén G, Hamsten A, Wiman B. Comparison of plasminogen activator inhibitor activity and antigen in plasma samples. Clin Chim Acta 1987; 169: 189–96.

20
Plasminogen activity

P. J. GAFFNEY

INTRODUCTION

Plasminogen is present in plasma as a proenzyme with respect to its major catalytic activity, namely the hydrolysis of fibrin and other components in blood. Other activities of plasminogen (e.g. its binding to fibrin, histidine-rich glycoprotein, HRGP, and α_2-antiplasmin) are partly or fully expressed in plasma by the proenzyme form and will not be discussed further here. The measurement of the plasminogen molecule in plasma has presented difficulties for many years due to its presence in plasma as a proenzyme and the interference of a number of plasmin inhibitors (notably α_2-antiplasmin) with the measurement of the activated form of the proenzyme, namely plasmin. Plasma plasminogen levels can be measured directly or indirectly. Indirect methods are based on the activation of the inactive plasminogen by streptokinase (SK) or urokinase (UK) to active plasmin which, being a proteolytic enzyme, can be assayed using a variety of methodologies and substrates. The substrates most commonly used have been gelatin[1], fibrinogen–fibrin[2-5], casein[6-10] and esters of arginine and lysine[11-14]. Further details of methods and substrates for the assay of plasmin have been reviewed[15]. Most direct assay methods for plasminogen are based on its affinity for a plasminogen antiserum and have been reported in the literature[16-20]. A listing of some of the assays, with references, is given in Table 20.1.

INDIRECT METHODS

Determination of plasminogen in plasma by an indirect method requires the removal or inactivation of the antiplasmins in the plasma. This can be done by acidification[2,9] and by precipitation with ammonium sulphate[17] or acetone[30]. These procedures remove the antiplasmins in the supernatant and

155

Table 20.1   Indirect and direct methods of plasminogen assay

Direct	
1. Affinity chromatography	Zolton et al.[21]
2. Haemagglutination inhibition	Ludlam and Das[22]
3. Immunoelectrophoresis	Ganrot and Nilehn[16]
4. Latex flocculation	Wu et al.[20]
5. Radial immunodiffusion	Storiko[23]
6. Radioimmunoassay	Rabiner et al.[18]
7. Amidolytic (SK-plgn complex)	Friberger et al.[24]
Indirect	
1. Caseinolytic	Remmert and Cohen[6]*
2. Esterolytic	Troll et al.[11]
3. Fibrinolytic (clot lysis)	Berg et al.[25]
4. Fibrinolytic (plate assay)	Wolf[26]
5. Fluorescence	Bell et al.[27]
	Pochron et al.[28]
6. Spectrophotometric	Smith et al.[29]

* Many workers have since extended and modified this method particularly, and others in this table. The references are intended to provide the source of the original or definitive method.

the precipitate is reconstituted and assayed as plasmin, following an appropriate activation procedure. It is the influence of this plasminogen activation procedure on the resultant plasmin activity which is the greatest problem in all indirect assays of plasminogen. Much of the problem relates to near-impossibility of fully activating all the plasminogen to active plasmin without plasmin autolysis (Figure 20.1). The dynamic molecular balance between plasminogen, plasminogen intermediate (PLG-i), active plasmin and inactivate plasmin renders it difficult to convert all the plasminogen to active plasmin without some digestion of the active site L-chain. In fact it has been suggested[31] that the indirect assay of plasminogen in plasma from the viewpoint of tedium and accuracy is somewhat incompatible with the requirements of routine laboratory practice.

DIRECT ASSAYS

Table 20.1 lists some direct assays, with appropriate references should details of these be required. Since the level of plasminogen in plasma is reasonably constant (~ 0.1 mg/ml plasma) and since the normal level is high compared with other components of haemostasis, methods of great sensitivity (e.g. radioimmunoassay, latex flocculation and haemagglutination inhibition) seem unnecessary. Thus the most practical and quantitative methods are those which can be applied to most components of blood which are present in reasonably large amounts, namely, radial immunodiffusion using some modification of the procedure of Mancini et al.[35] and the immunoelectrophoretic or 'rocket' procedure[36]. Since these are described in many textbooks it is necessary here only to emphasize their simplicity and reproducibility. Obviously the only problem in these assays is that denatured plasminogen and degraded forms of plasminogen will be measured as biologically intact

PLASMINOGEN ACTIVITY

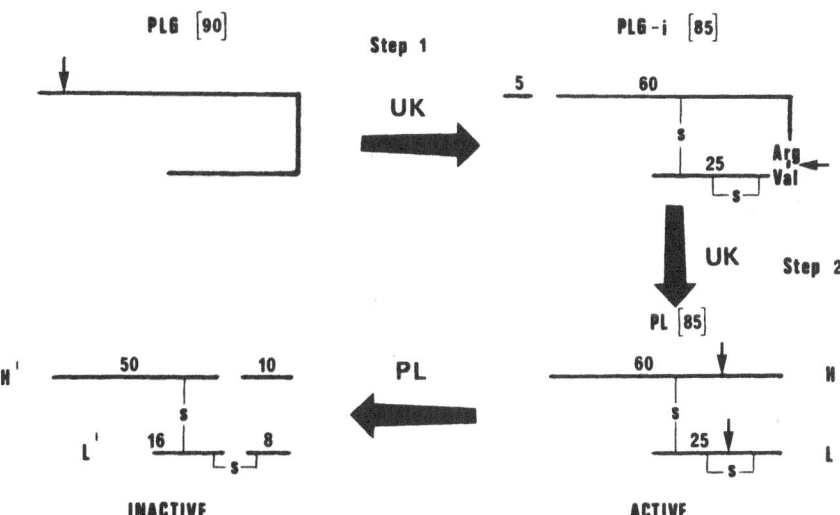

Figure 20.1 Schematic representation of the two-step activation of plasminogen followed by the autodigestive step from active to inactive plasmin. This scheme was compiled from data reported elsewhere[32-34]. PLG, PLG-i, PL and UK denote plasminogen, plasminogen intermediate, plasmin and urokinase. The numbers in brackets and numbers above the polypeptide chains (denoted by straight lines) are molecular weights $\times 10^{-3}$. Small arrows denote the approximate locations at which urokinase cleaves plasminogen to form an intermediate and finally plasmin. H and L denote the heavy and light chains of active plasmin, and H' and L' are their digested equivalents in the auto-digested inactive form of plasmin. A token number of disulphide bonds (S) is shown to explain the total loss of only 5000 MW peptides during the activation of plasminogen, and the molecular weights of the subunits show more significant changes. Step 1 shows the loss of 5000 MW peptide material during the formation of plasminogen intermediate, step 2 shows the cleavage of an arginylvalyl bond to form the two disulphide-bonded subunits of active plasmin, and plasmin converts active plasmin to an inactive form by the cleavage of the light and heavy chains, most probably at their C-terminal ends. (Taken from ref. 31)

molecules. The user must assess the clinical situation of the patient whose plasma is being assayed before a judgement can be made concerning the suitability of these assays.

Fortunately one method which can questionably be described as direct and yet measures functional activity has been developed[37]. This depends on the fact that a streptokinase–plasminogen (SK–plgn) complex can hydrolyse the presumed plasmin-specific chromogenic substrates S-2251 (Kabi Diagnostica, Sweden) and Chromozym-PL (Pentapharma, Switzerland). Since this complex is only poorly inhibited by α_2-antiplasmin and other plasma inhibitors it is possible to convert all the plasminogen in plasma to the SK–plgn complex following a 10-min incubation time. The complex, as measured by the hydrolysis of chromogenic substrate, is a direct reflection of the level of plasminogen in the test plasma. This assay obviates the problems of plasminogen activation referred to above and has allowed plasminogen assays to be conducted in plasma with some degree of confidence. This assay, using reagents from Kabi Diagnostica and KabiVitrum, was used in the ECAT studies (ECAT Assay Procedures Book no. 2).

Although a slight inhibition of the SK–plgn complex by excess SK has been reported[38] this does not affect the validity of assays for plasminogen when comparing one plasma with another. Purified plasminogen preparations are affected more by this inhibition, and this is probably the cause of the non-parallelism found when plasma plasminogen is compared in a dose–response manner with a purified glutamic acid–plasminogen (glu–plgn) standard (Figure 20.2). It was found[31] essential to maintain a constant plgn/SK ratio during the dose–response analysis of test and standard preparations of plasminogen (Figure 20.3). Thus while recommending this procedure as the only reliable direct plasma plasminogen assay certain precautions have to be taken when calibrating the assay using the glu–plgn standard. Problems have been reported when this type of assay is applied to patient plasma samples, notably patients with DIC and elevated fibrin degradation products[39,40] and patients with elevated levels of fibrinogen associated with ischaemic heart disease[41]. The fact that fibrinogen has been shown to enhance the enzymatic activity of the SK–plgn complex[35] has been used to obviate these effects and avoid an overestimation of plasminogen levels in the plasma of patients with DIC and elevated levels of fibrinogen. The assay to be described below was initially designed for the assay of plasminogen in plasma using a calibrated standard for glu–plgn. Due to the effect of fibrinogen and fibrin degradation products on the activity of the SK–plgn complex on chromogenic substrates we recommend that the purified plasminogen standard should be used in the presence of 1.0 mg/ml of plasminogen-free fibrinogen which is incorporated into buffer A below to give buffer B. Recommended details of the assay procedure are given below.

DETAILS OF RECOMMENDED DIRECT ASSAY OF PLASMINOGEN IN PLASMA

When streptokinase (SK) is added to a solution of plasminogen (i.e. plasma) a SK–plgn complex is formed in which the active site of the complex is exposed to such an extent that it can hydrolyse the chromogenic substrate H-D-Val-Leu-Lys-pNA (S-2251) releasing the yellow chromophore p-nitroaniline (pNA). An alternative chromogenic substrate known as Chromazym PL (Pentopharm, Basle, Switzerland) can be used to detect the complex. The activity of the activator complex on S-2251 is not affected by the fibrinolytic inhibitors in plasma, notably α_2-antiplasmin. If the amount of SK added to the sample is in excess of the plasminogen present, then an equimolar complex (SK–plgn) is formed, the amount of which is determined by the quantity of plasminogen. Thus under conditions of excess SK the rate of pNA production is a direct reflection of the amount of plasminogen in the sample. The pNA production can be followed by a recorder (initial rate method) or read after stopping the reaction with acetic acid (endpoint method). The final suggested outline of this assay given below was an amalgam from various reports in the literature [37,42,43].

PLASMINOGEN ACTIVITY

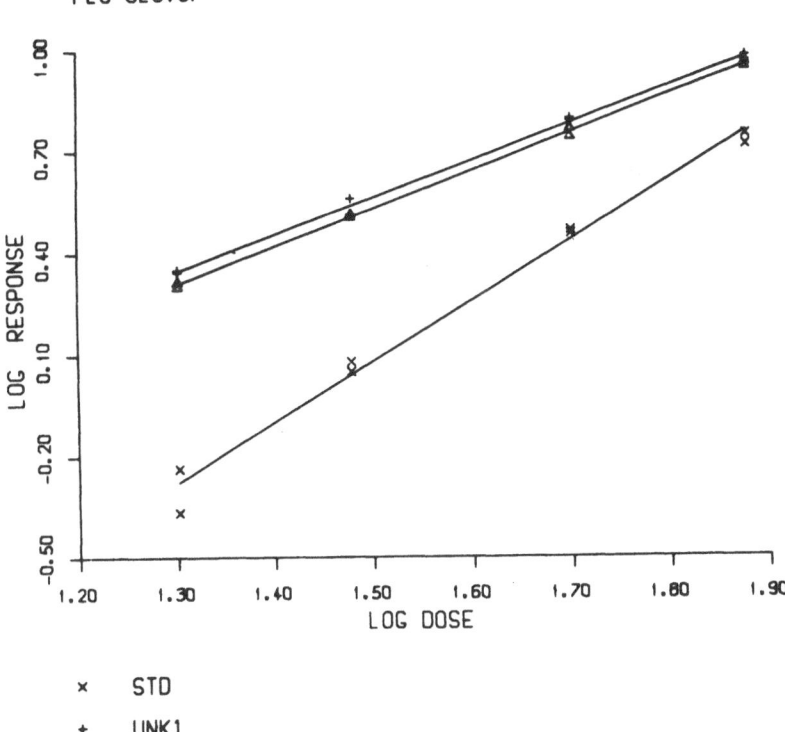

Figure 20.2   The log/log dose–response curves of the SK–plgn complexes formed in two plasmas (+, △) compared with that formed from purified glu–plgn (×). The response variable[31] is the rate (×10^{-3}s^{-1}) of optical density change of S-2251 at 405 nm

Equipment

Spectrophotometer (405 nm wavelength setting); semi-microcuvettes (1 ml); centrifuge; water bath (37 °C); stopwatch; disposable plastic test tubes.

Extra equipment for initial rate method: photometer cuvette housing at 37 °C; recorder.

Reagents

1. *Plasminogen-free fibrinogen*: freeze-dried reagent from IMCO (Sweden), reconstitute with distilled water to give a solution (2%) in 0.3 mol/L NaCl.
2. *Buffer A*: 50 mmol/L Tris HCl–12 mmol/L NaCl. Add 6.1 g Tris and 0.7 g NaCl to distilled water; adjust to pH 7.4 at room temperature with 1 mol/L HCl and make up to 1000 ml with distilled water. Stable for 2 months at 2–6 °C.
3. *Buffer B*: buffer A with plasminogen-free human fibrinogen added at 10.0 mg/ml.

159

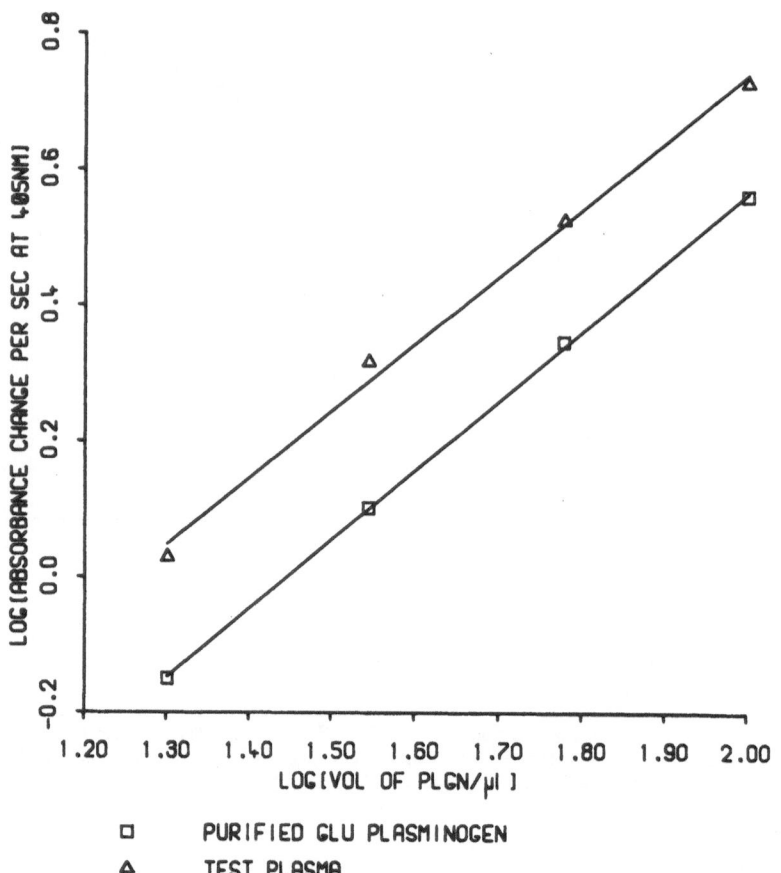

Figure 20.3 Comparison of the log/log dose–response curves of glu–plgn standard and normal test plasma using a consistent SK/plgn ratio in all dilutions[31]

4. *Chromogenic substrate*: alternatives: (a) H-D-Val-Leu-Lys-pNA, 2 HCl (S-2251); (b) Tos-Gly-Pro-Lys-pNA, HCl (Chromazym PL). Dissolve contents of manufacturer-supplied ampoule in sufficient distilled water to make a 3 mmolar solution. This is stable at 0–6 °C for 6 months. Add one part of this solution to eight parts buffer, mix well; this solution is subsequently referred to as the *substrate* and is 333 µmol/L. The substrate should be prepared on the day of assay and incubated at 37 °C.
5. *Activator* (*SK*): streptokinase (Kabikinase from Kabi AB, Stockholm, Sweden, or Streptase from Behringerke, Marburg, Germany) is reconstituted with distilled water to give a concentration of 10 000 i.u./ml.
6. *Plasminogen standard*: a glutamic acid–plasminogen (glu–plgn) standard (code 78/646) is available from the National Institute for Biological

Standards and Control, Potters Bar, Hertfordshire EN6 3QG, UK. It contains 10 units per ampoule and these units are the same as those defined by the second International Reference Preparation for plasmin. Reconstitute ampoule with 4 ml of buffer. This solution will be referred to as the *Standard* and contains 2.5 units per ml.

7. *Acetic acid (50%)*: this is used only in the endpoint method.

Assay procedure

Establishment of a calibration curve using the standard and the assay of the test plasma involves the same procedure and thus the construction of an assay curve for each will be described simultaneously.

1. To 100 μl of the standard and 100 μl of a 1:1 diluted test plasma add 400 μl of the activator (SK) solution and incubate at 37 °C for 10 min.
2. Dilute the SK-test plasma and SK-standard 1/1, 1/2, 1/3 and 1/4 with buffers A and B respectively.
3. To 100 μl of each dilution of the SK standard and SK test plasma add 900 μl of the chromogenic substrate solution and do this in a manner which is dependent on whether (a) continuous OD recording or initial rate is available or (b) the endpoint procedure is followed.
   (a) *Initial rate OD*: use disposable plastic cuvettes and stagger the addition of substrate so that there is time to follow the OD at 405 nm for about 1 min in a thermostatically controlled (37 °C) spectrophotometer. Each dilution of SK-standard and SK-test plasma will give a different OD/min and these data give a linear plot over a range of 0.2–2.0 units of plasminogen. The blank used in each case is distilled water.
   (b) *Endpoint*: add chromogenic substrate to each dilution of SK-standard and SK-test plasma in disposable plastic test tubes and incubate for exactly 3 min before stopping each reaction mixture by the addition of 100 μl of acetic acid (50%). Read the colour generated in each reaction mixture in a 1 ml plastic cuvette (light path = 1 cm). Use a blank made up of 900 μl of substrate, 100 μl of distilled water and 100 μl 50% acetic acid.

Note added Buffer B is recommended in DIC plasma samples; however, it is worthwhile to check the assay using buffer A only since the cost of the buffer B reagent is quite considerable.

Calculations

1. Plot the log OD against the log of the amount of plasminogen in units contained in each dilution measured. The graph is linear over a wide range (0.2–2.0 units/ml) (see Figure 20.3).
2. Each dilution of the test plasma generates an OD/min reading. The four separate values can be read from the calibration curve of the plasminogen standard. The average of these can be used to express the plasminogen concentration in plasma as units of plasminogen/ml.

References

1. Christensen LR, McLeod MC. A proteolytic enzyme of serum. Characterisation, activation with inhibitors. J Gen Physiol 1949; 28: 559–83.
2. Nilsson IM, Skanse B, Gydell K. Fibrinolysis in Boeck's sarcoid. Acta Med Scand 1957; 159: 463–70.
3. Lassen M. The estimation of fibrinolytic components by means of the lysis time method. Scand J Clin Lab Invest 1958; 10: 384–9.
4. Kowalski E, Kopec M, Niewiarowski S. An evaluation of the euglobulin method for the determination of fibrinolysis. J Clin Pathol 1959; 12: 215–18.
5. Vignal A, Blatrix C, Steinbuch M. Fibrinogen free of plasminogen as substrate for fibrinolytic assays. Nature, Lond 1962; 193: 693.
6. Remmert LF, Cohen P. Partial purification and properties of a proteolytic enzyme of human serum. J Biol Chem 1949; 181: 431–48.
7. Alkjaersig N, Fletcher AP. Sherry S. The mechanism of clot dissolution by plasmin. J Clin Invest 1959; 38: 1086–95.
8. Derechin M. The assay of human plasminogen with casein as substrate. Biochem J 1961; 78: 443–8.
9. Hedner U, Nilsson IM. Determination of plasminogen in human plasma by a casein method. Thromb Diath Haemorrh 1965; 14: 545–61.
10. Johnson AJ, Kline DL, Alkjaersig N. Assay methods and standard preparations for plasmin, plasminogen and urokinase in purified systems, 1967–1968. Thromb Diath Haemorrh 1969; 21: 259–72.
11. Troll W, Sherry S, Wachman J. The action of plasmin on synthetic substrates. J Biol Chem 1954; 208: 85–93.
12. Kline DL, Fishman JB. Plasmin. The humoral protease. Ann NY Acad Sci 1957; 68: 25–36.
13. Lassen M. The esterase activity of the fibrinolytic system. Biochem J 1958; 69: 360–6.
14. Roberts PS. Measurement of rate of plasmin action on synthetic substrates. J Biol Chem 1958; 232: 285–91.
15. Heimburger N. Plasminogen assay. A review and evaluation of various methods. In: Davidson, Samama M, Desnoyers, eds. Progress in chemical fibrinolysis and thrombolysis, vol. 1. New York: Raven Press, 1975; 173–9.
16. Ganrot PO, Nilehn JE. Immunochemical determination of human plasminogen. Clin Chim Acta 1968; 22: 335–40.
17. Hedner U, Nilsson IM. Comparison between a direct and indirect method for determining plasminogen. Thromb Diath Haemorrh 1971; 26: 289–94.
18. Rabiner SF, Goldfine ID, Hart A. Radioimmunoassay of human plasminogen and plasmin. J Lab Clin Med 1969; 74: 265–73.
19. Wu KK, Jacobsen CD, Hoak JC. Highly sensitive method for the assay of plasminogen. J Lab Clin Med 1973; 81: 484–8.
20. Wu KK, Jacobsen CD, Hoak JC. Assay of plasminogen using latex flocculation. Proc Soc Exp Biol Med 1973; 144: 391–3.
21. Zoltan RP, Mertz ET, Russell HT. Assay of human plasminogen in plasma by affinity chromatography. Clin Chem 1972; 18: 654–7.
22. Ludlam CA, Das PC. Plasminogen assay by haemagglutination inhibition technique. J Clin Pathol 1971; 24: 136–42.
23. Storiko K. Normal values for 23 different human plasma proteins determined by single radial immunodiffusion. Blut 1968; 6: 200–8.
24. Friberger P, Knos M, Gustavsson S, Aurell L, Claeson G. Methods for determination of plasmins, antiplasmin and plasminogen by means of substrate S-2251. Haemostasis 1978; 7: 138–45.
25. Berg W, Korsan-Bengtsen K, Ygge J. Determination of plasminogen in human plasma by the lysis time method. Thromb Diath Haemorrh 1966; 16: 1–17.
26. Wolf P. Modification of the fibrin plate for measurement of the components of the fibrinolytic system. Thromb Diath Haemorrh 1968; 20: 50–65.
27. Bell PJ, Dziobowski CT, Englert ME. A sensitive fluorometric assay for plasminogen, plasmin and streptokinase. Anal Biochem 1974; 61: 200–8.

28. Pochron SP, Mitchell GA, Albareda I, Huseby RM, Gargiulo RJ. A fluorescent substrate assay for plasminogen. Thromb Res 1978; 13: 733–9.
29. Smith RE, Bissell ER, Mitchell AR, Pearson KW. Direct photometric or fluorometric assay of proteineases using substrates containing 7-amino-4-trifluoromethylcoumarin. Thromb Res 1980; 17: 392–402.
30. Brakman P. Fibrinolysis. A standardized fibrin plate method and a fibrinolytic assay of plasminogen. Amsterdam: Scheltema & Holkema, 1967.
31. Gaffney PJ. Standardisation of plasminogen assays. Haemostasis 1988; 18 Suppl. 1: 47–60.
32. Rickli EE, Otavsky UI. Release of an N-terminal peptide from human plasminogen during activation with urokinase. Biochim Biophys Acta 1973; 295: 381–4.
33. Walther PJ, Steinman HM, Hill RL, McKee PA. Activation of human plasminogen by urokinase. Partial characterization of a preactivation peptide. J Biol Chem 1974; 249: 1173–81.
34. Wiman B, Wallen P. Activation of human plasminogen by an insoluble derivative of urokinase. Eur J Biochem 1973; 36: 25–31.
35. Mancini G, Carbonara AO, Heremans JF. Immunochemical quantitation of antigens by single radial immunodiffusion. Immunochemistry 1965; 7: 261–4.
36. Laurell CB. Quantitative estimation of proteins by electrophoresis in agarose gel containing antibodies. Anal Biochem 1966; 15: 45–9.
37. Friberger P, Knos M. Plasminogen determination in human plasma. In: Scully MF, Kakkar VV, eds. Chromogenic peptide substrates: chemistry and clinical usage. Edinburgh: Churchill Livingstone, 1979; 128–40.
38. Gaffney PJ, Philo RD. Measurement of some haemostatic components using biological and amidolytic assays. In: Davidson JF, Nilsson IM, Astedt B, eds. Progress in fibrinolysis, vol. 5. Edinburgh: Churchill Livingstone, 1981; 196–202.
39. Soria C, Soria J, Bertrand O, Dunn F, Samama M, Bachmann F. The amidolytic activity of the SK-plasminogen complex is enhanced by a potentiator which is generated in the presence of vascular plasminogen activator – role of fibrin degradation products. Thromb Haemostas 1982; 47: 193–6.
40. Gram J, Jespersen J. A functional plasminogen assay utilising the potentiating effect of fibrinogen to correct for the overestimation of plasminogen in pathological plasma samples. Thromb Haemostas 1985; 53: 255–9.
41. Gram J, Munkvad S, Jespersen J. Elevated plasma concentrations of fibrinogen assay cause an overestimation of functional plasminogen. Thromb Haemostas 1989; 61: 154.
42. Gaffney PJ, Philo RD. A commentary on new methodology in haemostasis using chromogenic substrates. In: Fareed J, Mesmore HL, Fenton JW, Brinkhous KM, eds. Perspectives in haemostasis. New York: Pergamon Press, 1981; 405–17.
43. Kabi Diagnostica Information Pamphlet. S-2251: Determination of plasminogen in plasma.

21
α_2-Antiplasmin activity

C. KLUFT

INTRODUCTION

The glycoprotein, α_2-antiplasmin, is a serine protease inhibitor of molecular weight 65–70 kD, present in plasma[1] in a concentration of approximately 1 µmol/L. The protein is synthesized in the liver and has a catabolism corresponding to a plasma half-life of about 2.5 days[2,3]. The inhibitor occurs in blood in two molecular forms: a plasminogen-binding (PB) and a non-plasminogen-binding (NPB) form[4]. On average the ratio[5] PB:NPB is 2:1.

The PB form is a very fast-acting plasmin inhibitor; NPB reacts 50–100 times more slowly[6-8]. The PB form of α_2-antiplasmin is responsible for the rapid plasmin inactivation observed in plasma. The assay principle of the 'immediate plasmin inhibition test', IPIT[9-11] is designed principally to detect the rapid inhibition in plasma and predominantly to report on the level of PB α_2-antiplasmin.

PRINCIPLE

The assay involves two reactions:

(a) Reaction of α_2-antiplasmin (AP) in diluted plasma with a known excess of plasmin

$$\text{AP} + \text{Plasmin} \rightleftharpoons \text{AP-plasmin} + \text{plasmin}$$
$$\text{(excess)} \qquad\qquad\qquad \text{(free)}$$

(b) Determination of the free plasmin by its amidolytic activity on a synthetic tripeptide chromogenic substrate (p-nitroanilide (pNA) release detected at 405 nm)

$$\text{Plasmin} + \text{chromogenic substrate} \rightarrow \text{pNA}$$
$$\text{(free)}$$

165

The rate of PNA release is compared to similar data of a calibration curve constructed by using different dilutions of pooled plasma standard. The content of the pooled plasma standard is set at 100% or 1 arbitrary U/ml.

EQUIPMENT

1. A recording spectrophotometer with a thermostated cuvette holder and the ability to measure at 405 nm (range 0–0.5; paper speed of recorder: 50 mm/min).
2. A water bath for 37 °C.
3. Ultra microcuvettes for 200–250 µl.
4. Stopwatch.

REAGENTS

1. *Tris buffer.* 50 mmol/L Tris buffer, pH 7.4 (at 25 °C) containing 110 mmol/L NaCl, 1.4 g/L Carbowax 6000 and 0.01% (v/v) Tween 80.
2. *Plasmin substrate stock.* D-Val-L-Leu-Lys-*p*-nitroanilide (S-2251, Kabi Diagnostica, Mölndal, Sweden). D-Val-Leu-Lys-pNA (19 mg) is dissolved in 10 ml distilled (preferably sterile) water to give a final concentration of 3.5 mmol/L. If not contaminated by microorganisms the solution can be stored refrigerated at about +5 °C, otherwise it should be stored frozen (−20 °C). Prior to use, the substrate solution should, after thawing, be kept in ice water for 1 h.
3. *Plasmin stock solution.* Plasmin is dissolved in 2 mmol/L HCl containing 50% (v/v) glycerol and 5 g/L polyethylene glycol (Carbowax) 6000 to a final concentration of 0.075–0.1 µmol/L (between 0.125 and 0.175 casein units/ml). This should correspond to an OD/min between 0.135 and 0.160 (1 cm pathway) in the test. The solution is stored in aliquots at −20 °C. Prior to use, the solution should be kept in ice water for 1 h.
4. *Fifty per cent acetic acid.*
5. Pooled citrated plasma for the calibration curve is obtained by mixing platelet-poor citrated plasma from 15–20 healthy volunteers and stored frozen, or alternatively is obtained from commercial sources, e.g. CTS-standard plasma from Behringwerke AG, Marburg, Germany.
6. *Quality control plasma.* Commercially available from Behringwerke AG, Marburg, Germany (CTS control plasma N labelled, 96% AP; CTS control plasma Pl labelled, 66% AP), Kabi Diagnostica, Mölndal, Sweden (Control plasma Kabi Normal, Control plasma Kabi Abnormal), Organon Teknika BV, Turnhout, Belgium (verify normal citrate) and Diagnostica Stago, Franconville, France (Stachrom Antiplasmin Control).
7. *Sample*: platelet-poor citrated plasma. No serum.

INITIAL RATE METHOD

1. *Adjustment of plasmin activity.* Add 120 µl Tris buffer to a small prewarmed polystyrene tube, followed by 40 µl of chromogenic substrate stock. Mix

and place in 37 °C water bath for 2–4 min. Add 40 µl of plasmin stock, mix immediately and transfer to prewarmed microcuvette. Record OD changes at 405 nm; assays are preferably in triplicate. Plasmin activity should be in the appropriate range (OD change per minute: 0.135–0.160), otherwise adjust.

2. *Construction of calibration curve.* Pooled normal plasma or commercially available standard plasma is diluted with Tris buffer to 25%, 50%, 75%. The six-point calibration curve is made with 2 µl of 0%, 25%, 50%, 75%, 100% and 2.5 µl (= 125%) plasma (or prediluted samples at expense of added buffer). See assay below. The points are determined in triplicate and the calibration curve is checked for quality (see Pitfalls).

3. *Assay.* Add 120 µl Tris buffer to a small prewarmed polystyrene tube, followed by 40 µl of chromogenic substrate stock and 2 µl test plasma (or prediluted plasma at expense of added buffer). Mix and place in 37 °C water bath for 2–4 min. Add 40 µl of plasmin stock, mix immediately and transfer to a prewarmed microcuvette. Record OD changes at 405 nm; assays are preferably in triplicate.

4. *Quality control.* (a) Include control plasma sample(s) in each assay run. (b) Measure every 30 min the 75% dilution of the calibration samples. With the manual method the within-run coefficient of variation (CV) is, in our hands, around 4% – in agreement with reported experiences[10]. For automated performance the between-run CV can be kept at low values around 3–5%[12–14].

5. *Calculation of the results.* The activity of α_2-antiplasmin in the test sample can be expressed as a percentage of the concentration in the calibration plasma (100%) by comparing the changes in OD 405 with the standard curve.

ENDPOINT METHOD

The initial rate method described above can be replaced by 'an endpoint' method in which the plasmin activity is measured over a given fixed time period. The measurement is started with the addition of plasmin and the plasmin activity is quenched by the addition of acetic acid after exactly 120 s incubation at 37 °C. The amount of product formed in that period is measured at 405 nm against buffer in a spectrophotometer. A sample blank is needed if the plasma is opaque, or if the bilirubin concentration exceeds 100 µmol/L.

Procedure

Fifty per cent acetic acid (20 µl) is added exactly 120 s after the addition of plasmin. Other additions are performed as described for the initial rate assay.

VARIATIONS IN PLASMA CONCENTRATION OF α_2-ANTIPLASMIN

In normal individuals, aged between 20 and 50 years and sex ratio approximately 1, α_2-antiplasmin activity assayed with the IPIT showed, in our laboratory, a narrow range: $104 \pm 11\%$ (SD), $n = 71$, range 85–139% without differences between males and females. This compared well with another estimation of the range (80–136%, $n = 90$)[15]. Very similar methods consistently show a narrow normal range for α_2-antiplasmin activity with a standard deviation of 9% in a meta-analysis in 1982 ($n = 265$)[10] and with SDs of 17% ($n = 50$)[16] and 15–17% ($n = 100$)[13] in some other reports.

The lower limit of the normal range allows a clear distinction of heterozygotes for α_2-antiplasmin deficiency from normals and normal family members[17-19]. The upper limit resembles that used by others (120–140%)[20] (see above). α_2-Antiplasmin is an acute-phase reactant[5,21,22] and can be found to be elevated to about 130–140% of normal.

Elevated α_2-antiplasmin has been observed in some cases with thrombotic complications[15,20,23,24] and in cases with type II hyperlipoproteinemia[25] and progressive renal failure[26].

Reduced plasma levels of α_2-antiplasmin activity can occur due to congenital deficiencies type I and II[27]. Acquired deficiencies are known for thrombolytic therapy, liver diseases, nephrotic syndrome, disseminated intravascular coagulation, amyloidosis, leukaemia (especially acute promyelocytic leukaemia[16,28]), L-asparaginase therapy[29], the postoperative period[22] and extracorporeal circulation[27]. In some cases the reduction might involve inactivation by elastase[16,28,30].

PITFALLS

1. *Quality of plasmin.* The rapid interaction between plasmin and the PB-α_2-antiplasmin requires a second site interaction between the two molecules which requires in plasmin an intact function of the site. As reported for some types of plasmin preparations[31], plasmin can lose functional integrity of this site, and lose its suitability for the assay. Presently, most commercially available plasmin preparations are suitable, but outdated material may gradually contain larger proportions of degraded plasmin. The presence of substantial amounts of degraded plasmin is observed as a deviation of the calibration curve at higher inhibition levels. It is chosen to work only in an area of 0–50% inhibition of plasmin, thus allowing for 50% degraded plasmin before problems in the assay arise.

2. *Stability of plasmin during assay runs.* Stability of the plasmin working solution during the assay is possible only when the described procedures are strictly adhered to. Occasionally, in practice of assay runs of several hours, a drift in activity is still observed. To recognize this a dilution of the calibration/standard plasma should be analysed every $\frac{1}{2}$ h. In principle the blank plasmin activity could be followed; however, the assay of blank plasmin activity may carry other problems (see pitfall 4). We therefore prefer to use the above procedure.

3. *Viscosity of the plasmin solution.* It should be recognized that it is technically demanding to reproducibly pipette the viscous plasmin solution.

4. *Effect of plasma on chromogenic substrate*. Plasma proteins can influence the solubility state of certain chromogenic substrates, notably H-D-Val-Leu-Lys-pNA. To replace plasma proteins in the blank assay, addition of non-ionic detergents provide a solution[14,32,33].

5. *Spontaneous activity of plasma on chromogenic substrate*. In clinical samples such as after recent activation of fibrinolysis, plasmin captured by α2-macroglobulin may occur in plasma. Other enzymes active on the chromogenic substrate may also occur. Enzymes captured by α2-macroglobulin retain significant activity on chromogenic substrates[34]. The spontaneous activity of plasma should be subtracted from the recorded activities in the assay, and can be assayed itself in the described procedure replacing plasmin by buffer.

6. *Activation* in vitro. During and shortly after thrombolytic therapy, high levels of thrombolytics occur in collected plasma samples. Activation of plasminogen can continue *in vitro*, also at 0 °C, and can artificially reduce α2-antiplasmin activity[35]. Additions to blood and plasma of PPACK[36] or GGACK[37] for inactivation of t-PA and u-PA, respectively, do not disturb assay of α2-antiplasmin activity[38].

OTHER METHODS

1. *Technical variations of the IPIT*. The IPIT in our hands shows a satisfactory specificity for α2-antiplasmin (only $<5\%$ residual activity in homozygous deficient cases[17,19]) and reasonable but not absolute specificity for the PB form of α2-antiplasmin. We determined a contribution of 14% of the NPB form of α2-antiplasmin[5,39]. Technical variations in the method include the use of a reversed scheme of addition of plasmin and chromogenic substrate including a consequent 20–60 s preincubation of plasmin with the diluted plasma. Several different chromogenic substrates are in use[40]. Commercially available methods generally use the reversed scheme of additions (CoaTest Antiplasmin, Stachrom-Antiplasmin, Chromostrate-α2-antiplasmin assay, Berichrom-α2-antiplasmin). The reversed addition scheme and preincubation allows, especially at 25 °C[41], a larger contribution of α2-macroglobulin to the assay[10]. This contribution of α2-macroglobulin can be nullified by preincubation of plasma with methylamine[42].

2. *Immunochemical methods* (radial and electroimmunodiffusion, enzyme immunoassays) assay both molecular forms of α2-antiplasmin. It should be recognized that these methods are complicated by the occurrence of differences in titre of antisera for the PB and NPB forms[39]. Correlations between activity and antigen methods can accordingly be rather good[42,43], but may also be poor[13], depending upon the antibodies used.

3. *Functional aspects of α2-antiplasmin*. (a) Binding to fibrin[44]. During coagulation, part of the α2-antiplasmin becomes bound to fibrin through the action of activated factor XIIIa. This binding involves about 35% of the PB-form of α2-antiplasmin (or 20% of the total α2-antiplasmin) and is negligible for the NPB form. This binding can be determined by the difference between plasma and serum (or clotted plasma) in the content

of α_2-antiplasmin. This should preferably be assayed with the IPIT, since only the PB form binds to fibrin. (b) Binding to plasminogen. Binding to plasminogen can be evaluated with plasma samples using a modified crossed immunoelectrophoresis method[5].

References

1. Wiman B. Human α_2-antiplasmin. Methods Enzymol 1981; 80: 395–408.
2. Collen D, Wiman B. Turnover of antiplasmin, the fast-acting plasmin inhibitor of plasma. Blood 1979; 53: 313–24.
3. Knot EAR, Drijfhout HR, Ten Cate JW, De Jong E, Iburg AHC, Kahlé LH, Grijm R. α_2-Plasmin inhibitor metabolism in patients with liver cirrhosis. J Lab Clin Med 1985; 105: 353–61.
4. Clemmensen I. Different molecular forms of α_2-antiplasmin. In Collen D, Wiman B, Verstraete M, eds. The physiological inhibitors of coagulation and fibrinolysis. Amsterdam: Elsevier/North-Holland, 1979; 131–6.
5. Kluft C, Los P, Jie AFH, Van Hinsbergh VWM, Vellenga E, Jespersen J, Henny C. The mutual relationship between the two molecular forms of the major fibrinolysis inhibitor α_2-antiplasmin in blood. Blood 1986; 67: 616–22.
6. Wiman B, Collen D. On the kinetics of the reaction between human antiplasmin and plasmin. Eur J Biochem 1978; 84: 573–8.
7. Wiman B, Boman L, Collen D. On the kinetics of the reaction between human antiplasmin and a low-molecular-weight form of plasmin. Eur J Biochem 1978; 87: 143–6.
8. Petersen LC, Clemmensen I. Kinetics of plasmin inhibition in the presence of synthetic tripeptide substrate. Biochem J 1981; 199: 121–7.
9. Teger-Nilsson AC, Friberger P, Gyzander E. Determination of a new rapid plasmin inhibitor in human blood by means of a plasmin specific tripeptide substrate. Scand J Clin Lab Invest 1977; 37: 403–9.
10. Friberger P. Chromogenic peptide substrates. Their use for the assay of factors in the fibrinolytic and the plasma kallikrein-kinin systems. Scand J Clin Lab Invest 1982; 42 suppl. 162: 41–7.
11. Gallimore MJ, Amundsen E, Aasen AO, Larsbraaten M, Lyngaas K, Svendsen L. Studies on plasma antiplasmin activity using a new plasmin specific chromogenic tripeptide substrate. Thromb Res 1979; 14: 51–60.
12. Jespersen J, Sidelmann J. Individual levels of plasma α_2-antiplasmin and α_2-macroglobulin during the normal menstrual cycle and in women on oral contraceptives low in oestrogen. Thromb Haemostas 1983; 50: 581–5.
13. Dick W, Cullmann W. Automatisierung eines neuen amidolytischen Verfahrens zur α_2-Antiplasmin-Bestimmung im Plasma. Lab Med 1983; 7: 51–4.
14. Jespersen J, Gram J, Sidelmann J. An amidolytic assay of α_2-antiplasmin using a centrifugal analyser. In: Davidson JF, Donati MB, Coccheri S, eds. Progress in fibrinolysis, VII. Edinburgh: Churchill Livingstone, 1985; 193–7.
15. Engesser L. Thrombophilia. Disorders of blood coagulation and fibrinolysis. Thesis, Leiden University, 1988.
16. Aoki N. Hemostasis associated with abnormalities of fibrinolysis. Blood Rev 1989; 3: 11–17.
17. Kluft C, Vellenga E, Brommer EJP, Wijngaards G. A familial hemorrhagic diathesis in a Dutch family: an inherited deficiency of α_2-antiplasmin. Blood 1982; 59: 1169–80.
18. Miles LA, Plow EF, Donnelly KJ, Hougie C, Griffin JH. A bleeding disorder due to deficiency of α_2-antiplasmin. Blood 1982; 59: 1246–51.
19. Kluft C, Nieuwenhuis HK, Rijken DC, Groeneveld E, Wijngaards G, Van Berkel W, Dooijewaard G, Sixma JJ. α_2-Antiplasmin Enschede: dysfunctional α_2-antiplasmin molecule associated with an autosomal recessive hemorrhagic disorder. J Clin Invest 1987; 80: 1391–400.
20. Kluft C, Leebeek FWG. α_2-Antiplasmin and thrombosis: results of a questionnaire. Fibrinolysis 1988: 2, suppl. 2: 47–8.
21. Matsuda M, Wakabayashi K, Aoki N, Morioka Y: α_2-Antiplasmin inhibitor is among acute-phase reactants. Thromb Res 1980; 17: 527–32.

22. Kluft C. Fibrinolytic shut-down after surgery. In: Sawaya R, ed. Fibrinolysis and the central nervous system. Philadelphia, PA: Hanley & Belfus, 1990; 127–40.
23. Brommer EJP, Gevers Leuven JA, Kluft C, Wijngaards G. Fibrinolytic inhibitor in type II hyperlipoproteinaemia. Lancet 1982; 1: 1066.
24. Ratnoff OD. The role of haemostatic mechanisms. Clin Haematol 1981; 10: 261–81.
25. Lowe GDO, Stromberg P, Forbes CD, McArdle BM, Lorimer AR, Prentice CRM. Increased blood viscosity and fibrinolytic inhibitor in type II hyperlipoproteinaemia. Lancet 1982; 1: 472.
26. Gordge MP, Faint RW, Rylance PB, Kluft C, Nield GH. Abnormal fibrinolysis in progressive renal failure due to a reduction in circulating tissue plasminogen activator. Br J Haematol 1988; 69: 133.
27. Saito H. α₂-Plasmin inhibitor and its deficiency states. J Lab Clin Med 1988; 112: 671–8.
28. Avvisati G, Ten Cate JW, Sturk A, Lamping RJ, Petti MC, Mandelli F. Acquired α₂-antiplasmin deficiency in acute promyelocytic leukaemia. Br J Haematol 1988; 70: 43–8.
29. Vellenga E, Kluft C, Mulder NH, Wijngaards G, Nieweg HO. The influence of L-asparaginase therapy on the fibrinolytic system. Br J Haematol 1984; 57: 247–54.
30. Brower MS, Harpel PC. Proteolytic cleavage and inactivation of α₂-plasmin inhibitor and C1-inactivator by human polymorphonuclear leukocyte elastase. J Biol Chem 1982; 257: 9849–54.
31. Kluft C, Traas DW, Jie AFH, Hoegee-de Nobel E. The suitability of various plasmin preparations for the functional assay of α₂-antiplasmin in plasma. Thromb Haemostas 1982; 48: 320–4.
32. Kluft C, Wijngaards G, Jie AFH, Groeneveld E. Appropriate milieu for the assay of α₂-antiplasmin activity with chromogenic substrates. Haemostasis 1985; 15: 198–203.
33. Jespersen J, Gram J, Sidelmann J. Modification of the immediate plasmin inhibition assay to secure linearity of the reference curve with the chromogenic substrate S-2251. Thromb Haemostas 1984; 51: 298.
34. Gyzander E, Teger-Nilsson AC. Activity of the α₂-macroglobulin-plasmin complex on the plasmin specific substrate H-D-Val-Leu-Lys-p-nitroanilide. Thromb Res 1980; 19: 165–75.
35. Rijken DC, Seifried E, Barrett-Bergshoeff MM, Dooijewaard G. Plasminogen activation at low temperatures in plasma samples containing therapeutic concentrations of tissue-type plasminogen activator or other thrombolytic agents. Thromb Haemostas 1990; 64: 47–52.
36. Seifried E, Tanswell P. Comparison of specific antibody, D-Phe-Pro-Arg-CH₂Cl and aprotinin for prevention of in vitro effects of recombinant tissue-type plasminogen activator on haemostasis parameters. Thromb Haemostas 1987; 58: 921–6.
37. Lijnen HR, Van Hoef B, Collen D. Differential reactivity of Glu-Gly-Arg-CH₂Cl, a synthetic urokinase inhibitor, with single-chain and two-chain forms of urokinase-type plasminogen activator. Eur J Biochem 1987; 162: 351–6.
38. Oethinger MD, Seifried E. In vitro effects of urokinase – prevention by different inhibitors. Thromb Haemostas 1990; 64: 402–6.
39. Kluft C, Jie AFH, Los P, Dooijewaard G, Traas DW. Expression of the two forms of α₂-antiplasmin in functional and immunochemical assays. In: Davidson JF, Bachmann F, Bouvier CA, Kruithof EKO, eds. Progress in fibrinolysis, VI. Edinburgh: Churchill Livingstone, 1983; 386–7.
40. Svendsen LG, Fareed J, Walenga JM, Hoppensteadt D. Newer synthetic peptide substrates in coagulation testing: some practical considerations for automated methods. Semin Thromb Hemostas 1983; 9: 250–62.
41. Naito K, Aoki N. Assay of α₂-plasmin inhibitor activity by means of a plasmin specific tripeptide substrate. Thromb Res 1978; 12: 1147–56.
42. Matsuda T, Ogawara M, Miura R, Seki T, Matsumoto T, Teramura Y, Nakamara K. Selective determination of α₂-plasmin inhibitor activity in plasma using chromogenic substrate. Thromb Res 1984; 33: 379–88.
43. Aoki N, Yamanaka T. The α₂-plasmin inhibitor levels in liver diseases. Clin Chim Acta 1978; 84: 99–105.
44. Sakata Y, Aoki N. Cross-linking of α₂-plasmin inhibitor to fibrin by fibrin-stabilizing factor. J Clin Invest 1980; 65: 290–7.

22
Plasmin-α_2-antiplasmin complexes

E. HATTEY, M. HAUMER, A. BINDER and B. R. BINDER

INTRODUCTION

α_2-Antiplasmin is the most important plasmin inhibitor. Its rapid reaction with plasmin results in the formation of an inactive complex composed of one molecule of each component. Two steps are involved in this process: first, a reversible complex is formed between the lysine-binding site of plasmin and complementary sites on the carboxyterminal end of the α_2-antiplasmin molecule. In a second step an irreversible complex is generated associated with the cleavage of a peptide bond in the inhibitor[1]. During activation of plasminogen to plasmin and plasmin action an equilibrium exists between formation of plasmin-α_2-antiplasmin complexes, occurring preferentially in the fluid phase and binding and action of plasmin on the fibrin surface. Bound to fibrin, plasmin is protected against inhibition by α_2-antiplasmin[2,3]. However, whenever fibrin is completely dissolved the plasmin liberated from the fibrin surface is immediately complexed by α_2-antiplasmin[2,3].

Whenever fibrin forms in the circulation, this process will be accompanied by activation of the fibrinolytic system because of the well-known effects of fibrin on tissue plasminogen activator (t-PA)[4,5]. Plasmin generated thereby will in part become complexed with α_2-antiplasmin, leading to increased levels of plasmin-α_2-antiplasmin (PAP) complexes. Such increased levels of PAP complexes have therefore been found in many circumstances in which fibrin formation is increased as in thrombophilia, hypercoagulability, disseminated intravascular coagulation, endotoxic shock, leukaemia, liver diseases, nephrotic syndromes or after major surgery[6-24]. Even in plasma after venous occlusion in most cases increased plasmin-α_2-antiplasmin levels have been found consistent with increased fibrin formation and increased levels of tissue plasminogen activator in the venous occlusion plasma[25].

While in all cases mentioned above only a limited increase of PAP levels is observed, thrombolytic therapy leads by extensive activation of the

173

fibrinolytic system to a massive plasmin formation in the fluid phase and maximal PAP complex formation[26]. Non-fibrin-specific plasminogen activators such as streptokinase or urokinase can cause complete consumption of plasmin inhibitors, resulting in an increased bleeding tendency due to plasminaemia. The plasmin action is therefore no longer restricted to its specific substrate, fibrin, but extended to non-specific substrates such as fibrinogen and other coagulation factors.

Determination of plasmin−α_2-antiplasmin complexes on the one hand can therefore serve as indicative for general plasminaemia during hyperfibrinolytic states with fibrinogen and α_2-antiplasmin consumption and possible bleeding tendency; on the other hand, slightly increased levels of plasmin−α_2-antiplasmin complexes are indicative for ongoing thrombus formation and thrombus dissolution, as in the case of thrombophilia.

METHODS OF ASSAY

To determine PAP complexes, several test methods have been published including two-dimensional immunoelectrophoresis, latex assay, RIA and more recently ELISA systems.

Initially a latex agglutination assay for determination of PAP complexes was introduced by Plow et al.[27] with rather low sensitivity. Then a two-dimensional electrophoresis was described using the different mobilities of free and complexed α_2-antiplasmin[6,28]. This method was still not sensitive enough and rather time-consuming, and not applicable for a larger number of samples. Employing polyclonal antisera raised against plasmin B-chain, α_2-antiplasmin complexes, an RIA was developed by Wiman et al.[29] thereby avoiding recognition of intact plasminogen or plasmin. But intact α_2-plasmin could still be detected together with the PAP complex, though to a much lesser extent.

A great advance was the development of the double sandwich technique used in the ELISA systems. Since then, several methods have been developed, either utilizing an antibody against antiplasmin as a catching antibody, and an antibody against the enzyme as detecting antibody, or vice-versa[30−33]. Harpel[30] first published a sensitive assay with a polyclonal antibody against α_2-antiplasmin as catching antibody and POX-labelled Fab fragments against plasminogen as detecting system, whereby the Fab fragments are preferred to whole antibodies to reduce unspecific binding of plasminogen and other plasma proteins to immunoglobulins. Other ELISA systems were described by Holvoet et al.[31] and Mimuro et al.[33] employing either two monoclonal antibodies against either part of the complex or one polyclonal and one monoclonal antibody. Most recently a liposome immune lysis assay (LILA) was introduced by Hosoda et al.[34]. The ELISA or LILA test systems described up to now have, however, certain limitations because of interference of the abundant amounts of uncomplexed α_2-plasmin or plasminogen with the rather low concentrations of PAP complex. Another disadvantage arises from the fact that, to our knowledge, none of these test systems are commercially available or easy to prepare for everyone, at least not in Europe; the PAP kit TD-80C, quoted in the literature from Teijin, Tokyo, Japan, is at present not for sale in Europe (personal communication, Teijin managing director, April 1991).

We therefore recommend in this paper a test system which is very sensitive and more specific for PAP complexes by employing a monoclonal antibody against the neoantigen in the PAP complex as catching antibody. Furthermore, the test can easily be performed because all components are commercially available.

Test principle

The test described here is a solid-phase enzyme immunoassay in which MPW7AP, a specific monoclonal antibody directed against the neoantigen of the PAP complex, is adsorbed on plastic microtitre plates. During incubation with test samples PAP complexes are selectively bound, and after washing away unbound material the complexes are detected by MPW2PG POX, a peroxidase-labelled monoclonal antibody against the kringle 1–3 region of the plasmin(ogen) part of the complex. Quantification of labelled antigen–antibody conjugates is achieved by ABTS, a chromogenic substrate for peroxidase.

Material and equipment

1. Flat-bottom microtitre plates (96-well) with high binding capacity (e.g. NUNC immunoplate maxisorp 4-93454 or GREINER ELISA plates (no. 655061), plate sealers (e.g. COSTAR 3095).
2. ELISA reader for 405 nm and 492 nm wavelength (e.g. Anthos reader 2001, Zinsser, Austria).
3. Antibody to PAP neoantigen MPW7AP and antibody to kringle 1–3 region of plasmin(ogen) POX-labelled, MPW2PG POX (Technoclone, Vienna, Austria).
4. PAP complex standard plasma and PAP complex depleted plasma (Technoclone, Vienna, Austria).
5. ABTS [2-2′ azinobis(3-ethylbenz-thiazolinesulphonic acid)] from Boehringer Mannheim, Germany.
6. Aprotinin (Trasylol^R) from Bayer, Leverkusen, Germany.
7. 2-[Ethylmercury(π)-thio]-benzoic acid sodium salt (Thimerosal^R) 818957, Merck, Germany.
8. Polyoxyethylene sorbitan monooleate (Tween 20) P 13 79, Sigma USA.
9. Serum albumin bovine, purified (BSA) ORHO 20/21, Behring, Germany.
10. Benzamidinium chloride 820122, Merck, Germany.

Solutions

Coating buffer: 1.59 g $Na_2CO_3.10H_2O$, 2.93 g $NaHCO_3$, 100 mg thimerosal with distilled water to 1L, pH 9.6.

Coating solution: 20 µg/ml MPW7AP in coating buffer; 100 µl/well.

Phosphate buffered saline (PBS): 8 g NaCl, 0.2 g KH$_2$PO$_4$, 1.44 g Na$_2$HPO$_4$.2H$_2$O with distilled water to 1L, pH 7.4.

Washing buffer: PBS + 0.5% Tween 20.

Blocking solution: PBS + 1% BSA.

Dilution buffer 1 (DB1): PBS + 1% BSA + 2000 KIU/ml aprotinin + 20 mmol/L benzamidinium chloride or a specific inhibitor for t-PA, e.g. PPACK.

Dilution buffer 2 (DB2): DB1 + 1% PAP depleted plasma.

Dilution buffer 3 (DB3): DB1 + 10% PAP depleted plasma.

Detecting solution: 10 µg/ml MPW2PG POX in DB1; 100 µl/well.

Substrate buffer: 1.29 g citric acid monohydrate, 1.375 g Na$_2$HPO$_4$.2H$_2$O with distilled water to 100 ml, pH 4.0.

Substrate solution: 1 mg ABTS/ml solution + 1 µl H$_2$O$_2$ 30%/ml solution in substrate buffer; 100 µl/well.

Stop solution: 320 mg NaF/100 ml distilled water; 100 µl/well.

Stability of the reagents

Coating buffer and coated plates containing an antimicrobial substance are stable at 4 °C. Other protein-containing solutions and washing buffer should be prepared freshly or kept under sterile conditions to prevent microbial growth. Antibiotics should not be used in these cases, to avoid adverse reactions with the peroxidase.

Procedure

Preparation of plates

The wells of an ELISA plate are filled with 100 µl/well coating solution, preferably by use of a multichannel micropipette. The plate should remain covered with a self-adhesive plastic foil for at least 16 h at 4 °C but can also be stored that way for prolonged time. Before use, the plate is emptied and refilled with 100 µl/well of blocking solution and incubated for 1 h at 37 °C to block excessive reactive groups on the plate surface. For all incubation steps the plate remains covered with the plastic foil.

Sample preparation

Normal citrated or EDTA plasma can be used, but one should be aware that uninhibited plasminogen activators will lead to *in vitro* formation of PAP complexes. Especially in monitoring thrombolytic therapy, blood samples should always be collected into anticoagulants containing inhibitors, e.g. 2000 KIU/ml aprotinin + 20 mmol/L benzamidine final concentration.

The plasma samples are diluted 1:10 in DB1 for low concentrations and 1:100 for high concentrations of PAP complexes; 100 µg/well are needed, and at least duplicate determinations are recommended.

Standard preparation

PAP complex standard plasma is reconstituted with distilled water. Serial dilutions from 1:100 to 1:800 and blanks are prepared in DB3 for use with low PAP concentration samples and in DB2 for use with samples containing high PAP concentrations. 100 µl/well and duplicates are also necessary.

Washing of the plates

Between all incubation steps the plates are washed three times with approximately 300 µl/well washing buffer either manually or by use of an automatic plate washer. After each emptying step the plate is carefully tapped dry on absorbent paper towels.

Flow sheet of procedure

1. Coating of ELISA plates overnight at 4 °C.
2. Incubation with blocking solution 1 h at 37 °C.
3. Washing step.
4. Incubation of samples overnight at 4 °C.
5. Washing step.
6. Incubation with detecting solution 2 h at 37 °C.
7. Washing step.
8. Incubation with substrate solution 30 min at room temperature, protected from light.
9. Addition of stop solution.
10. Reading of the plate in an ELISA reader with 405 nm test wavelength and 492 nm reference wavelength within 2 h.
11. Plotting of standard values on linear scale and reading of sample values from the respective standard curve for high and low PAP concentrations; multiplication with the dilution factor.

Evaluation of results

For evaluation of the results, the reading of the samples is compared with those of a reference PAP complex preparation.

Standardization

Since plasmin–α_2-antiplasmin complexes are not easily prepared in a stable purified form – the complex is susceptible to proteolytic degradation and different epitopes might be generated whether the complex is formed in excess of plasmin or of inhibitor (1) – we decided to prepare PAP complexes directly in plasma and to calibrate them with PAP complexes generated from purified components. For this purpose citrated plasma was incubated with more than saturating concentrations of urokinase to produce maximum amount of plasmin–α_2-antiplasmin complexes. Thereafter the reaction was terminated by addition of benzamidine and Trasylol. The complexes so formed are stable either frozen at $-70\,^{\circ}$C or lyophilized at $4\,^{\circ}$C. To determine the actual amount of complexes in the standard plasma the readings in the ELISA assay were compared with those of PAP complexes generated from purified components. For this purpose plasmin was prepared freshly from purified Glu–plasminogen by incubation with urokinase bound to Sepharose and after removal of urokinase Sepharose the resulting plasmin activity was determined with S-2251 immediately and after 30 min incubation with purified α_2-antiplasmin at $37\,^{\circ}$C. The differences in plasmin activity represent the amount of PAP complexes formed (Figure 22.1).

Specificity

The described test is specific for plasmin–α_2-antiplasmin complexes and allows full plasma recovery provided the standard was diluted in PAP-depleted plasma in the same concentration as the plasma samples to be tested.

Difficulties, source of error, trouble-shooting

The major source of error in the PAP ELISA described lies in the preparation of samples and a possible *ex vivo* PAP complex formation. Therefore, care has to be taken to collect blood samples into a suitable inhibitor whenever plasminaemia or plasmin formation after blood collection is expected. See section 'Sample preparation'.

Sensitivity and normal values

In this assay the lower detection limit is 10 ng/ml in purified systems as well as in plasma.

PLASMIN–α₂-ANTIPLASMIN COMPLEXES

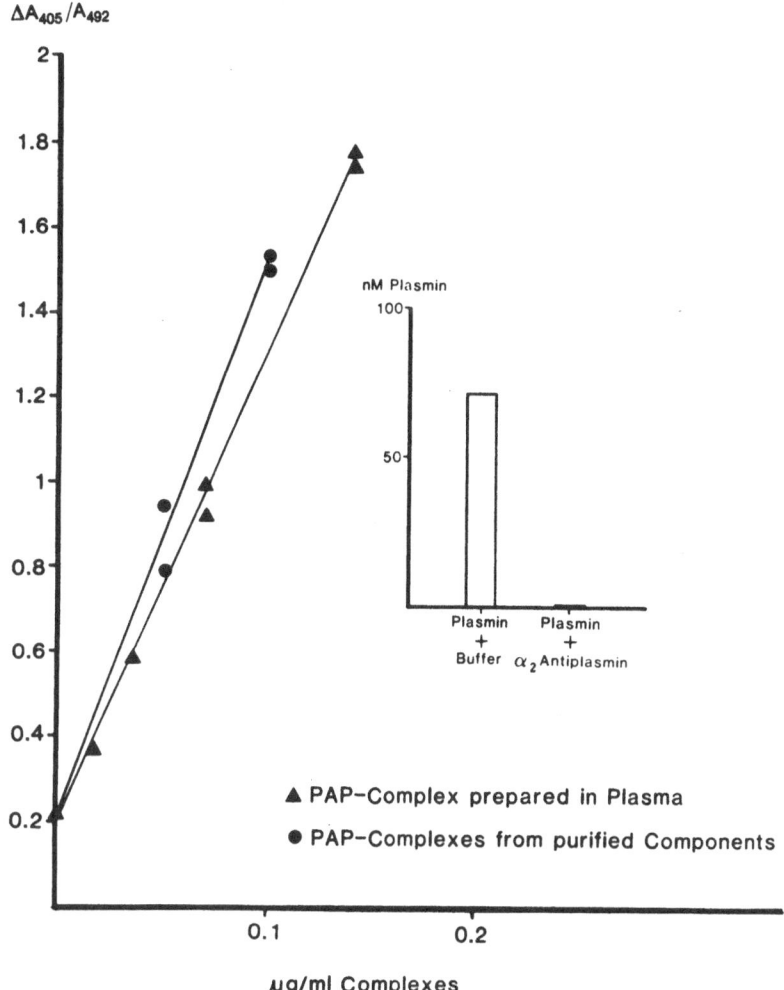

Figure 22.1 Comparison of PAP complexes prepared in plasma with PAP complexes from purified components. In the insert the amidolytic determination of plasmin activity from freshly prepared plasmin incubated with buffer or without excess α_2-antiplasmin is shown. From the differences in plasmin activity (plasmin inhibited) the concentration of bound complexes is calculated.

1. Normal values: in a normal control population mean PAP values in citrated plasma are 152 ± 72 ng/ml and 132 ± 72 ng/ml in EDTA plasma; in serum samples PAP values are mostly increased.
2. Pathological values: thrombolytic therapy results in PAP plasma values of > 800 ng/ml. In patients with coronary heart disease treated successfully by percutaneous transluminal coronary angiography (PTCA) PAP values were found to be increased 12 months thereafter (Figure 22.2).

179

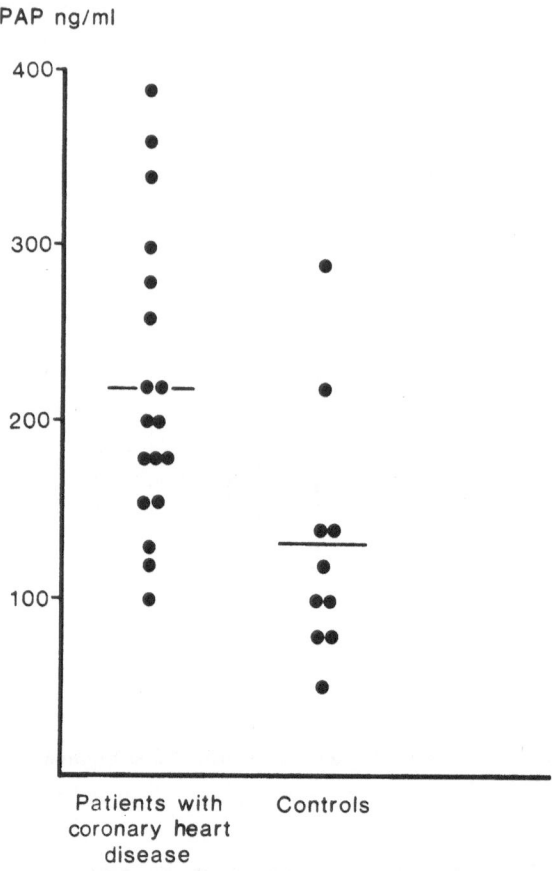

Figure 22.2   PAP complexes in controls and patients with coronary heart disease

Control and calibration procedures

There is no internationally recognized PAP standard available at the moment; therefore, standardization can be done by comparison with a commercially available reference plasma with given PAP content or in a similar manner as described in the Standardization Section.

Comparison with data from other studies

See Table 22.1.

Table 22.1 Comparisons with data obtained by others*

	Normal plasma	Fully activated plasma
Latex agglutination[27] (only titre)	1:4	1:512
Crossed immunelectrophoresis[28], semiquantitative (0 to + + +)	0	+ + +
Radioimmunoassay[29], lower limit 1.5 µg/ml	0–2 µg/ml	n.d.
ELISA[30] anti-α_2-AP as catching antibody antiplasminogen F(ab)$_2$ as detecting antibody	4.1–3.5 fmol/ml plasmin equivalent	177.6 fmol/ml plasmin equivalent
ELISA[7,32] † antiplasminogen (polyclonal) catching antibody anti-α_2-AP monoclonal as detecting antibody	0.2 ± 0.1 µg/ml	n.d.
LILA[34] (same system as above)	0.8 ± 0.4 µg/ml	n.d.
ELISA[35–37] ‡ antineoantigen monoclonal as catching antibody antiplasminogen monoclonal as detecting antibody	152 ± 72 ng/ml	> 1 µg/ml

* No direct comparison of test systems could be performed because of a lack of availability of several reagents
† This system corresponds to a PAP kit commercially available from Teijin
‡ This system corresponds to a PAP kit commercially available from Technoclone

References

1. Wiman B. Human α_2-antiplasmin. Methods Enzymol 1981; 80: 395–408.
2. Sakata Y, Aoki N. Significance of cross-linking of α_2-antiplasmin inhibitor to fibrin in inhibition of fibrinolysis and in hemostasis. J Clin Invest 1982; 69: 536–542.
3. Aoki N, Harpel PC. Inhibitors of the fibrinolytic enzyme system. Sem Thromb Hemostas 1984; 10: 24–41.
4. Hoylaerts M, Lijnen DC, Collen D. Kinetics of the activation of plasminogen by human tissue plasminogen activator. J Biol Chem 1982; 257: 2912–19.
5. Beckmann R, Geiger M, Binder BR. Plasminogen activation by tissue plasminogen activator in the presence of stimulating CNBr fragment FCB-2 of fibrinogen is a two-phase reaction. J Biol Chem 1988; 263: 7176–80.
6. Booth NA, Bennett B. Plasmin–α_2-antiplasmin complexes in bleeding disorders characterized by primary or secondary fibrinolysis. Br J Haematol 1984; 56: 545–56.
7. Takahashi H, Tatewaki W, Wada K, Yoshikawa A, Shibata A. Thrombin and plasmin generation in patients with liver disease. Am J Hematol 1989; 32: 30–5.
8. Suffredini AF, Harpel PC, Parrillo JE. Promotion and subsequent inhibition of plasminogen activation after administration of intravenous endotoxin to normal subjects. N Engl J Med 1989; 320: 1165–72.
9. Negoro N, Kanayama Y, Takeda T, Fujisawa M, Okamura M, Inoue T. Plasminogen activation in plasma of patients with systemic lupus erythematosus. Rheumatol Int 1989; 8: 273–7.
10. Matsuda T, Asakura H, Ito K, Saito M, Jokaji Y, Uotani C, Kumabashiri I. Changes in levels of t-PA and alpha-2PI-plasmin complex in plasmin with patients with DIC. Thromb Res 1988; Suppl. 8: 143–51.

11. Egbring R, Seitz R. Improved prognosis of fulminant hepatic failure (FHF) after plasma derivative replacement therapy. Enhanced proteolysis of hemostatic proteins confirmed by proteinase-inhibitor complexes determination. Z Gastroenterol 1990; 28: 104–9.
12. Mellbring G, Dahlgren S, Wiman B. Plasma fibrinolytic activity in patients undergoing major abdominal surgery. Acta Chir Scand 1989; 151: 109–14.
13. Takahashi H, Hanano M, Takizawa S, Tatewaki W, Shibata A. Plasmin-alpha-2-plasmin inhibitor complex in plasma of patients with disseminated intravascular coagulation. Am J Hematol 1988; 28: 162–6.
14. Galloway MJ, Mackie MJ, McVerry BA. Circulating plasmin–antiplasmin complexes in acute leukaemia. Clin Lab Haematol 1983; 5: 243–51.
15. Burtin P, Chavanel G, Andre-Bougaran J, Gentile A. The plasmin system in human adenocarcinomas and their metastases. A comparative immunofluorescence study. Int J Cancer 1987; 39: 170–8.
16. Velasco F, Torres A, Andres P, Martinez F, Gomez P. Changes in plasma levels of protease and fibrinolytic inhibitors induced by treatment in acute myeloid leukemia. Thromb Haemostas 1984; 52: 81–4.
17. Teufelsbauer H, Proidl S, Wolner E, Vukovich Th. Activation of hemostasis during cardiopulmonary bypass: Evidence for thrombin mediated hyperfibrinolysis (In press).
18. Mellbring G, Dahlgren S, Reiz S, Wiman B. Fibrinolytic activity in plasma and deep vein thrombosis after major abdominal surgery. Thromb Res 1983; 32: 575–84.
19. Takahashi H, Tatewaki W, Wada K, Hanano M, Shibata A. Thrombin vs. plasmin generation in disseminated intravascular coagulation associated with various underlying disorders. Am J Hematol 1990; 33: 90–5.
20. Kawakami M, Kawagoe M, Harigai M, Hara M, Hirose T, Hirose W, Norioka K, Suzuki K, Kitani A, Nakamura H. Elevated plasma levels of alpha 2-plasmin inhibitor-plasmin complex in patients with rheumatic diseases. Possible role of fibrinolytic mechanism in vasculitis. Arthritis Rheum 1989; 32: 1427–33.
21. Tomiya T, Hayashi S, Ogata I, Fujiwara K. Plasma alpha 2-plasmin inhibitor-plasmin complex and FDP-D-dimer in fulminant hepatic failure. Thromb Res 1989; 53: 253–60.
22. Saito M, Asakura H, Uotani C, Jokaji H, Kumabashiri I, Matsuda T. Quantitative estimation of elastase-alpha 1-proteinase inhibitor (E-alpha 1-PI) complex in leukemia: marked elevation in cases of acute promyelocytic leukemia. Thromb Res 1989; 53: 163–71.
23. Mellbring G, Dahlgren S, Wiman B. Prediction of deep vein thrombosis after extensive abdominal operations by the quotient between plasmin–alpha 2-antiplasmin complex and fibrinogen concentration in plasma. Surg Gynecol Obstet 1985; 161: 339–42.
24. Speiser W, Pabinger-Fasching I, Kyrle PA, Kapiotis S, Kottas-Heldenberg A, Bettelheim P, Lechner K. Hemostatic and fibrinolytic parameters in patients with acute myeloic leukemia: activation of blood coagulation, fibrinolysis and unspecific proteolysis. Blut 1990; 61: 1–5.
25. Wiman B, Mellbring G, Ranby M. Plasminogen activator release during venous stasis and exercise as determined by a new specific assay. Clin Chim Acta 1983; 127: 279–88.
26. Urano T, Kamiya T, Sakaguchi S, Takada Y, Takada A. Fibrinogenolysis and fibrinolysis in normal volunteers and patients with thrombosis after infusion of urokinase. Thromb Res 1985; 39: 145–55.
27. Plow EF, de Cock F, Collen D. Immunochemical characterization of the plasmin–antiplasmin system. Basis for the specific detection of the plasmin–antiplasmin complex by latex agglutination assays. J Lab Clin Med 1979; 93: 199–209.
28. Booth NA, Bennett B. Plasmin–α2-antiplasmin complex as an indicator of in vivo fibrinolysis. Br J Haematol 1982; 50: 537–41.
29. Wiman B, Jacobsson L, Andersson M, Mellbring G. Determination of plasmin-α_2-antiplasmin complex in plasma samples by means of a radio-immunoassay. Scand J Clin Lab Invest 1983; 43: 27–33.
30. Harpel PC. α2-plasmin inhibitor and α2-macroglobulin-plasmin complexes in plasma. Quantitation by an enzyme-linked differential antibody immunosorbent assay. J Clin Invest 1981; 68: 46–55.
31. Holvoet P, Lijnen HR, Collen D. A monoclonal antibody specific for Lys-plasminogen. J Biol Chem 1985; 260: 12106–11.
32. Aoki N, Takenaga T, Hasegawa J, Oguma U, Sumi Y, Koike U, Suzuki H, Hosoda K.

Fundamental assessment of enzyme immunoassay kits for α_2 plasmin inhibitor (α_2PI) and α_2-PI-plasmin complex. Jpn J Clin Pathol 1987; 35: 1275–81.

33. Mimuro J, Koike Y, Sumi Y, Aoki N. Monoclonal antibodies to discrete regions in α2-plasmin inhibitor. Blood 1987; 69: 446–53.

34. Hosoda K, Yasuda T. Homogeneous immunoassay for α2 plasmin inhibitor (α_2PI) and α_2PI-plasmin complex. Application of a sandwich liposome immune lysis assay (LILA) technique. J Immunol Methods 1989; 121: 121–8.

35. Hattey E, Wojta J, Binder BR. Monoclonal antibodies against plasminogen and alpha-2-antiplasmin: binding to native and modified antigens. Thromb Res 1987; 45: 485–95.

36. Hattey E, Wojta J, Huber K, Binder BR. Development and evaluation of ELISA systems for determination of plasmin-alpha-2-antiplasmin (PIP) complexes in plasma. Fibrinolysis 1986; suppl. 1: A152.

37. Hattey E, Beckmann R, Krutisch G, Huber K. Evaluation of limited activation of the plasma fibrinolytic system during thrombolysis by rtPA. Fibrinolysis 1988; 2 suppl. 1: 2.

23
Plasma histidine-rich glycoprotein (HRG)

J. GRAM

INTRODUCTION

Histidine-rich glycoprotein (HRG) is a specific plasma protein, which binds reversibly to plasminogen via the lysine-binding sites. The binding of HRG to plasminogen decreases to about 50% the amount of free plasminogen available for fibrinolysis. Thus, HRG is considered to be a fibrinolysis regulatory protein.

Physiological role

HRG was originally purified by Heimburger and co-workers in 1972[1]. At that time no biological function of this protein was known, but more recently HRG has been demonstrated to be potentially involved in several biological functions, such as the homeostasis of divalent metal ions[2], the immunoresponse[3], the neutralization in plasma of heparin[4] and in the regulation of haemostasis[5].

   Like several other plasma proteins involved in haemostasis HRG has been supposed to be produced by the liver[6,7], but it has also been suggested that a main production site of HRG is bone-marrow megakaryocytes[8]. In plasma HRG is present in a native 75 000 MW form and a partially degraded 60 000 MW form. Both of these forms of HRG are involved in the regulation of haemostasis, which might be related to the following steps:

   release from and binding to platelets[8,9]
   fibrin polymerization[10]
   heparin neutralization[4]
   inhibition of fibrinolysis[11].

Particularly, the role of HRG in the inhibition of fibrinolysis has become of interest, because a defective fibrinolysis has been reported to play an important role in the evolution of arteriosclerosis[12], and arterial and venous thrombosis[5,13]. HRG binds to the lysine binding sites of glu–plasminogen with a K_d of about $1 \mu mol/L$[11,14]. *In vitro* experiments have definitely demonstrated that the binding of HRG to plasminogen reduces the adsorption of glu–plasminogen to fibrin, and thereby retards effective fibrinolysis[11].

Pathophysiological aspects

A variety of clinical conditions has been reported to be associated with deviations in plasma concentrations of HRG (Table 23.1).

Of most interest are conditions with elevated plasma concentrations of HRG, because these may potentially be involved in the pathophysiology of thrombotic disease. Recently, Engesser and co-workers reported their results of a family with thrombosis inherited during five generations[20]. The family was characterized by an increased risk of both arterial and venous thrombosis, which could exclusively be explained by high plasma concentrations of HRG, i.e. up to 180% of that in pooled normal plasma. This study illustrates that elevated plasma concentrations of HRG may increase the risk of both arterial and venous thrombosis. From a physiological point of view this is understandable, because elevated plasma concentrations of HRG decrease the concentrations of free plasminogen available for fibrinolysis. Also, patients with a congenital plasminogen deficiency are characterized by an increased risk of both arterial and venous thrombosis[23].

METHODS OF ASSAY

Histidine-rich glycoprotein was originally isolated as a 3.8 s α_2-glycoprotein with a molecular weight of 60 000[1], which is now considered to be a proteolytic derivative of a native molecule with a molecular weight[4] of 75 000. The partially degraded molecule is present in human plasma[11,17-19] in a concentration of about 1.8 μmol/L and conventional immunological techniques, such as radial immunodiffusion and immunoelectrophoresis, are sufficiently sensitive methods to determine human plasma concentrations reliably. So far, no convenient functional routine methods have been developed for the

Table 23.1 Decreased or increased concentrations in plasma of histidine-rich glycoprotein (HRG) in relation to pathological conditions

---

Decreased concentrations of HRG
    Thrombolytic therapy[15,16]
    Sepsis[17]
    Acute phase reactions[18,19]
    Liver cirrhosis[6,7]

Increased concentrations of HRG
    Familial thrombosis[20]
    Non-familial thrombosis[21,22]
    Leg vein thrombosis in myocardial infarction[18]

---

determination of HRG. Within the framework of ECAT immunoelectrophoresis is recommended as the official method.

Principle

The determination of the antigen concentration of HRG makes use of the well-known principle of single-dimension immunoelectrophoresis[24]. This assay involves the incorporation into agar gel of polyclonal IgG antiserum raised in rabbits against human HRG with a molecular weight of 60 000 (Behringwerke, Marburg). The antigen standards are applied along with the sample. The heights of the precipitin 'rockets' are plotted to establish a calibration curve, and the height of the sample precipitin 'rocket' is then converted to a concentration by use of the calibration curve.

MATERIALS

The general procedure for preparation of gels and performance of immunoelectrophoresis has been reviewed previously (see e.g. refs 24, 25).

Tris Barbital buffer (pH 8.8)

Trizma Base (Sigma, St Louis), 5.78 g; Sodium barbiturate (Merck, Darmstadt), 9.76 g; Barbituric acid (Merck, Darmstadt), 2.47 g; Distilled water containing 150 i.u. heparin (porcine mucosa, Leo Pharmaceuticals, Copenhagen), 1500 ml. Adjust to pH 8.8. Storage: $+4\,°C$. Stability: at $+4\,°C$, 6 months; at room temperature, 1 week.

Agarose 1% gel

Litex HSA (Litex, Copenhagen), 2.5 g; Tris-barbital buffer (pH 8.8), 250 ml. Storage: refrigerator in lots of 10 ml. Stability: at $+4\,°C$, 6 months.

HRG antiserum (Behringwerke)

Storage: refrigerator. Stability: expiration date on the vial.

Calibrator

Pool of platelet-poor K_3-EDTA (0.38 mol/L) plasma from at least 40 healthy volunteers. Exclude women who use OC. Storage: $-80\,°C$ in lots of 300 µl. Stability: at least 1 year.

Control

Pool of platelet-poor plasma (sodium citrate, $1 + 9$) collected from 10 volunteers. Storage: $-80\,°C$ in lots of 300 µl. Stability: at least 1 year.

Procedure

Prepare 1 mm gel plates after addition of 80 µl HRG antiserum to 20 ml agarose 1% to give a final antiserum concentration of 0.4% (v/v). Prepare the following calibrator solutions:

200%: 100 µl EDTA plasma + 300 µl isotonic NaCl
100%: 50 µl EDTA plasma + 350 µl isotonic NaCl
50%: 25 µl EDTA plasma + 375 µl isotonic NaCl
25%: 25 µl EDTA plasma + 775 µl isotonic NaCl

Dilute 50 µl sample specimen with 350 µl isotonic NaCl. Dilute 50 µl control specimen with 350 µl isotonic NaCl. Apply at the cathode 5 µl of calibrator, sample or control under a high voltage fall (50 V). Adjust voltage to 4.5 V/cm and run the electrophoresis for 18 h.

Evaluation of results

By the use of the calibrators described here the results will be expressed as percentages of the concentration in pooled normal plasma. However, it has repeatedly been reported that the antigen concentration of HRG in pooled normal plasma is 1.8 µmol/L[11,20,25]; hence it is possible by the use of this value to give an estimate of the patient plasma in SI units. The described procedure secures a linear calibration curve in the range of 0–200%

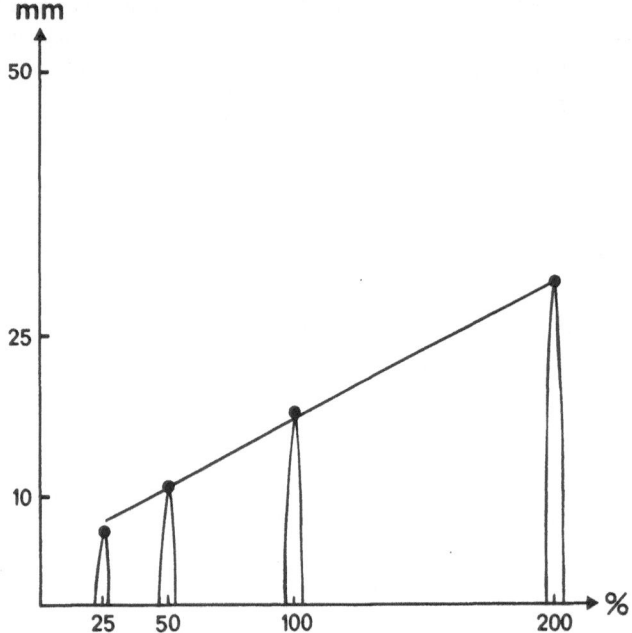

Figure 23.1 A calibration curve for histidine-rich glycoprotein (MW 60 000). Ordinate: Length of precipitin rockets. Abscissa: Concentrations of calibrator (a pool of normal plasma) in the range 25–200%

(Figure 23.1). Concentrations exceeding 200% should be further diluted and analysed in a new electrophoresis.

It should be noted that the determination immunologically of both plasminogen and HRG makes it possible to estimate the concentration of free plasminogen not bound to HRG. Histidine-rich glycoprotein is reversibly bound to plasminogen with a K_d of 1 µmol/L.

$$HRG + Plg \rightleftharpoons HRG*Plg$$
$$(a - x) \quad (b - x) \qquad (x)$$

$$\frac{(a - x) \times (b - x)}{x} = K_d (1 \, \mu mol/L)$$

In this equation a represents the concentration of total HRG; b represents the total concentration of plasminogen (Plg); x represents the calculated concentration of HRG complexed with plasminogen; and $b - x$ represents the concentration of free plasminogen not bound to HRG.

Normal values of HRG

Normal values are 50–150%.

Control and calibration

Due to the lack of well-characterized HRG control and calibration material, it is up to now necessary to use internal laboratory preparations. Histidine-rich glycoprotein in normal plasma stored at $-80\,°C$ is stable for at least 1 year. It might be advantageous to plot the control values in the Levey–Jennings control chart and use the principle of the Westgaard 'multi-rule shewhart chart' for quality control[26]. Such a procedure will give valuable information on both random error and systematically analytical bias.

References

1. Heimburger N, Haupt H, Kranz T, Bauder S. Humanserumproteine mit hoher Affinität zu Carboxymethylcellulose. II. Physikalischchemische und immunologische Charakterisierung eines histidine-reichen 3.8 S-α_2-Glycoproteins (CM-protein I). Hoppe Seyler's Physiol Chem 1972; 353: 1133–40.
2. Morgan WT. Interactions of the histidine-rich glycoprotein of serum with metals. Biochemistry 1981; 20: 1054–61.
3. Rylatt DB, Sia DY, Mundy JP, Parish CR. Autorosette inhibition factor: isolation and properties of the human plasma protein. Eur J Biochem 1981; 119: 641–6.
4. Lijnen HR, Collen D. Interaction of heparin with histidine-rich glycoprotein. Ann NY Acad Sci 1989; 556: 181–5.
5. Gram J. The haemostatic balance in groups of thrombosis-prone patients. With particular reference to fibrinolysis in patients with myocardial infarction. Thesis. Dan Med Bull 1990; 37: 210–34.
6. Gram J, Jespersen J, Ingeberg S, Bentsen KD, Back E. Levels of histidine-rich glycoprotein and plasminogen and the variation of free plasminogen in chronic liver disease. Thromb Res 1985; 39: 411–7.

189

7. Saito H, Goodnough LT, Boyle JM, Heimburger N. Reduced histidine-rich glycoprotein levels in plasma of patients with advanced liver cirrhosis. Am J Med 1982; 73: 179–82.
8. Leung LLK, Harpel PC, Nachman RL, Rabellino EM. Histidine-rich glycoprotein is present in human platelets and is released following thrombin stimulation. Blood 1983; 62: 1016–21.
9. Lerch PG, Nydegger UE, Kuyas C, Haerberli A. Histidine-rich glycoprotein binding to activated human platelets. Br J Haematol 1988; 70: 219–24.
10. Leung LLK. Interaction of histidine-rich glycoprotein with fibrinogen and fibrin. J Clin Invest 1986; 77: 1305–11.
11. Lijnen HR, Hoylaerts M, Collen D. Isolation and characterization of a human plasma protein with affinity for the lysine binding sites in plasminogen. Role in the regulation of fibrinolysis and identification as histidine-rich glycoprotein. J Biol Chem 1980; 255: 10214–22.
12. Astrup T. Fibrinolysis – an overview. In: Davidson JF, Rowan RM, Samama MM, Desnoyers PC, eds. Progress in chemical fibrinolysis and thrombolysis. Vol. 3. New York: Raven Press, 1978; 1–57.
13. Jespersen J. Pathophysiology and clinical aspects of fibrinolysis and inhibition of coagulation. Experimental and clinical studies with special reference to women on oral contraceptives and selected groups of thrombosis prone patients. Thesis. Dan Med Bull 1988; 35: 1–33.
14. Kluft C, Los P. Modified crossed immunoelectrophoresis to study with whole plasma the reversible complex formation of histidine-rich glycoprotein with plasminogen. Thromb Haemost 1988; 60: 411–4.
15. Lijnen HR, De Cock F, Collen D. Turnover of human histidine-rich glycoprotein in healthy subjects and during thrombolytic therapy. Thromb Res 1981; 23: 121–31.
16. Smith A, Nuiry I, Morgan WT. Proteolysis of histidine-rich glycoprotein in plasma and in patients undergoing thrombolytic therapy. Thromb Res 1985; 40: 653–61.
17. Lijnen HR, Jacobs G, Collen D. Histidine-rich glycoprotein in a normal and a clinical population. Thromb Res 1981; 22: 519–23.
18. Jespersen J, Gram J, Bach E. A sequential study of plasma histidine-rich glycoprotein and plasminogen in patients with acute myocardial infarction and deep vein thrombosis. Thromb Haemost 1984; 51: 99–102.
19. Saigo K, Yoshida A, Ryo R, Yamaguchi N, Leung LLK. Histidine-rich glycoprotein as a negative acute phase reactant. Am J Hematol 1990; 34: 149–50.
20. Engesser L, Kluft C, Briët E, Brommer EJP. Familial elevation of plasma histidine-rich glycoprotein in a family with thrombophilia. Br J Haematol 1987; 67: 355–8.
21. Samama M, Conard J, Castel-Gatey M, Horellou MH. Histidine-rich glycoprotein and deep vein thrombosis. In: Jespersen J, Kluft C, Korsgaard O, eds. Clinical aspects of fibrinolysis and thrombolysis. Esbjerg: South Jutland University Press, 1983; 163–73.
22. Engesser L, Kluft C, Juhan-Vague I, Briët E, Brommer EJP. Plasma histidine-rich glycoprotein and thrombophilia. Fibrinolysis 1988; 2/Suppl 2: 43–6.
23. Dolan G, Preston FE. Familial plasminogen deficiency and thromboembolism. Fibrinolysis 1988; 2/Suppl 2: 26–34.
24. Laurell C-B. Electroimmuno assay. Scand J Clin Invest 1972; 29/Suppl 124: 21–37.
25. Axelsen NH, Krøll J, Weeke B. A manual of quantitative immunoelectrophoresis. Methods and applications. Scand J Immunol 1973; 2/Suppl 1: 1–169.
26. Westgaard JO, Barry PL, Hunt MR, Groth T. A multi-rule shewhart chart for quality control in clinical chemistry. Clin Chem 1981; 27: 493–501.

24
Quantitative enzyme immunoassays for degradation products of fibrinogen (FgDP), fibrin (FbDP) and total of FgDP and FbDP (TDP)

W. NIEUWENHUIZEN

INTRODUCTION

Under normal physiological conditions the (low) activities of coagulation and fibrinolysis are balanced. It has long been recognized that the assessment of the products of these two opposing processes, i.e. fibrin and fibrin degradation products, may be of clinical and diagnostic value for the detection of possible disturbances in the haemostatic balance.

Both the conversion of soluble fibrinogen to insoluble fibrin and fibrin dissolution are multi-step processes that proceed via a series of intermediate products. In this paper some enzyme immunoassays will be described which can be used for the determination of fibrin(ogen) degradation products in plasma samples.

FORMATION OF FIBRIN(OGEN) DEGRADATION PRODUCTS

Formation of fibrinogen degradation products (fibrinogenolysis)

Under extreme disease conditions, but especially during thrombolytic therapy with streptokinase, the plasmin activity, generated in the circulation, may temporarily be incompletely inhibited by the natural plasmin inhibitors. Plasmin, the most important fibrinolytic enzyme, is in itself not fibrin-specific. It may also degrade other plasma proteins, including coagulation factors, e.g. fibrinogen.

When plasmin digestion of fibrinogen occurs, the first product which is formed is designated fragment X. Fragments X are slowly clottable and can be described as fibrinogen molecules from which about 60% of the length of both Aα-chains has been removed. From a single fragment X, one fragment Y and one fragment D are subsequently formed. Fragment Y is composed of one D- and one E-domain. Fragment Y will eventually be cleaved into one E- and one D-fragment.

Thus one fibrinogen molecule will yield two D-fragments and one E-fragment.

Formation of fibrin degradation products

Plasmin digestion of the different forms of fibrin proceeds via intermediate products, analogous to those described above for fibrinogen, since plasmin follows the same interdomainal cleavage pattern in fibrin as in fibrinogen.

Non-crosslinked desAA fibrin (fibrin I) will subsequently yield fragments X_I, Y_I, D, E_I and desAABB fibrin (fibrin II) will yield X_{II}, Y_{II}, D, E_{II}. The suffixes I and II denote the absence of FpA and of both FpA and FpB, respectively.

Crosslinked fibrins I and II consist of very long polymers of fibrin I and II, in which the subunits are covalently linked by isopeptide bonds. Plasmin will attack the fibrin subunits in these polymeric structures in a random order. This will result in smaller, soluble fragments of the original polymers, with a range of molecular weights[1,2]. These are collectively designated as X-oligomers[2-4]. Eventually, these X-oligomers can be digested to fragments of D-dimer, i.e. two covalently bound D-domains[1,2], and fragments E.

Serum samples should not be used

Even in disease states the blood concentrations of fibrin(ogen) derivatives will be low, as compared with the fibrinogen concentration, i.e. in the μg/ml range. For that reason, sensitive immunological methods such as enzyme immunoassays (EIA) or latex agglutination assays are required. Until relatively recently, only serum could be used as a sample, since the available polyclonal antibodies crossreact virtually completely with fibrinogen. Therefore, the latter had to be removed, e.g. by serum preparation. Well-known serum assays are the Thrombo-Wellcotest assay and the tanned red-cell haemagglutination inhibition assay[5]. Serum, however, is a notorious source of artifactual results, for example:

1. Incomplete clotting of the crossreacting fibrinogen may occur in cases of dysfibrinogenaemia; when a patient has been exposed to heparin[6] or when anticoagulating fibrinogen degradation products are present[7-9]. In polyclonal antibody-based serum assays this will inevitably lead to spuriously high or false-positive results. These can also result from partial lysis of the clot during serum preparation, not only in hyperfibrinolytic patients, but even in normal individuals[10].

2. Some degradation products will coagulate[8,11] or become adsorbed to the clot[10,12,13]. For that reason they will not be recovered in the serum, and false-negative or spuriously low results may be obtained.
3. During serum preparation, fibrinogen degradation products will lose their FpA. As a result they can no longer be discriminated from non-crosslinked fibrin degradation products, and primary fibrinogenolysis cannot be detected.
4. Serum can obviously not be used for the assessment of the products of ongoing coagulation in a patient.

The problems inherent in the use of serum could be avoided by using plasma. Only relatively recently, with the advent of monoclonal antibody technology, has it become possible to develop assays that can be performed with plasma samples, thus avoiding the serum artifacts mentioned above.

In the following paragraphs three of the new assays based on monoclonal antibodies (MoAb) will be described which can be performed with plasma samples, i.e. an assay specific for degradation products of fibrinogen (FgDP)[14-16]; an assay for fibrin degradation products (FbDP)[14,17] and an assay for the total of FgDP and FbDP (TDP)[10,14,15]. The three sandwich-type enzyme immunoassays (EIA) are manufactured by Organon Teknika, Boxtel, The Netherlands, and sold under the trade names Fibrinostika FgDP, Fibrinostika FbDP and Fibrinostika TDP, respectively. Other commercially available assays are summarized in Table 24.2.

PATHOPHYSIOLOGY

The clinical experience with the new assays is rapidly growing and fibrin(ogen) degradation products have been measured in plasma samples of patients with a variety of diseases.

The assays have been applied in (patho)physiological situations such as disseminated intravascular coagulation (DIC), deep venous thrombosis (DVT) and pulmonary embolism (PE), in pregnancy and (pre)eclampsia, in coronary artery disease and thrombolytic therapy, in liver disease and transplantation and in malignancies. For more detailed information the reader is referred to a review on this matter[18].

Fibrinolysis appears to be associated with (low grades of) fibrinogenolysis. The process of secondary fibrinolysis, as derived from FbDP levels, appears to predominate in deep venous thrombosis, pulmonary embolism, myocardial infarction and unstable angina. Thrombolytic therapy, especially with streptokinase, results in a pronounced fibrinogenolysis (primary fibrinolysis) as assessed by the levels of FgDP. The occurrence of an extensive fibrinogenolysis was also observed during orthotopic liver transplantation. Several diseases, such as DIC, malignancies and liver disease, exhibit both fibrinogenolysis and fibrinolysis secondary to an activated state of coagulation.

Plasma FbDP levels, as detected by EIA, reflect decreases in thrombus size and may be used to monitor efficacy of heparin treatment. Low initial values of FbDP are predictive of poor thrombus dissolution in patients with DVT following streptokinase or urokinase therapy. Elevated plasma levels of crosslinked fibrin degradation products have been measured during thrombolytic therapy of acute myocardial infarction. They are derived mainly from extracoronary sites and are non-predictive of recanalization following thrombolytic therapy.

Plasma fibrin degradation product levels are related to severity of liver cirrhosis. The observed increased fibrin(ogen) levels during normal and complicated pregnancy suggest that fibrinolysis is not necessarily depressed. The fibrinolytic system remains active in patients with malignancies, as demonstrated by elevated levels of D-dimers and FbDPs. The following guidelines for future studies are suggested. As mentioned in the introduction, a disturbance in the haemostatic balance will presumably be reflected in the products of both coagulation and fibrinolysis. In this chapter the focus has been on fibrin(ogen)olysis. Detection of fibrin(ogen) derivatives by the monoclonal antibody-based assays provides valuable information on haemostasis in several diseases. However, it is conceivable that more clinically relevant information can be obtained when the products of the two opposing processes, coagulation and fibrinolysis, are simultaneously measured. This possibility is available. Soluble fibrin, the product of an activated coagulation system, can also be assessed by EIA in plasma[19-21]. In the future, studies may be performed using a combination of an EIA for a coagulation product (i.e. soluble fibrin) and an EIA for a fibrinolysis product (i.e. FbDP or D-dimer).

Fibrinostika FgDP, principle and characteristics

The capture antibody in this EIA is a MoAb (FDP-14) specific for degraded forms of both fibrinogen and fibrin, i.e. it does not react with intact fibrin and fibrinogen[14]. When the test sample is incubated in the well of a microtitre plate coated with FDP-14 both FgDP and FbDP will be bound. The tagging antibody (Y18) in this EIA is specific for fibrinopeptide A-containing material[15]; it does not react with free fibrinopeptide A.

On the basis of the specificities of FDP-14 and Y18 we can conclude that the assay is specific for degradation products comprising fibrinopeptide A, i.e. FgDP[16].

Analysis of 42 healthy individuals in an outside laboratory showed an upper limit for FgDP of 250 ng FE/ml (FE = fibrinogen equivalent unit). This is an indication only, and each laboratory should determine its own normal range.

Fibrinostika FbDP

The capture MoAb of this EIA is FDP-14, i.e. the same as in Fibrinostika FgDP. However, the tagging MoAb is specific for FbDP. It is important to note that it does not discriminate between crosslinked and non-crosslinked FbDP. In that respect it is not comparable with the existing EIAs for D-dimer. The combination of the specificities of the capture and tagging antibodies in Fibrinostika FbDP make this EIA specific for FbDP[17].

Analysis of 42 healthy individuals in an outside laboratory showed an upper limit for FbDP of 310 ng FE/ml. This is an indication only, and each laboratory should determine its own normal range.

Fibrinostika TDP

The capture antibody, in this EIA also, is FDP-14. Thus, in the first step of this EIA both FgDP and FbDP are bound. The tagging antibody consists of a mixture of MoAbs used in Fibrinostika FgDP and Fibrinostika FbDP. This means that in Fibrinostika TPD both FgDP and FbDP (= TDP) are detected. The EIA has been published in a version in which polyclonal tagging antibodies were used[10].

The reproducibilities are given in Table 24.1. Analysis of 42 healthy individuals in an outside laboratory showed an upper limit for FgDP of 650 ng FE/ml. This is an indication only, and each laboratory should determined its own normal range. The specificities of the three Fibrinostika EIAs and some other commercially available EIAs are summarized in Table 24.2.

The procedures of the three Fibrinostika EIAs are virtually the same. The procedure for Fibrinostika FgDP is given in detail below.

Table 24.1 Reproducibility of Fibrinostika FgDP, FbDP and TDP; clinical samples (three runs in triplicate)

Sample*	CV (%) within-run for Fibrinostika			CV (%) between-run for Fibrinostika		
	FgDP	FbDP	TDP	FgDP	FbDP	TDP
1	15.7	4.2	11.0	19.3	10.8	27.2
2	7.0	5.0	9.3	12.5	14.8	30.8
3	8.1	6.7	8.8	14.0	18.3	4.2
4	3.3	3.7	1.9	8.9	21.5	15.5

* Concentration samples 1, 2, 3 and 4 used in:
  Fibrinostika FgDP 6785, 3176, 1341 and 257 ng FE/ml;
  Fibrinostika FbDP 8132, 5128, 1961 and 713 ng FE/ml;
  Fibrinostika TDP 9978, 5273, 1842 and 256 ng FE/ml, respectively

DETAILED SPECIFICS OF THE ASSAYS

Fibrinostika FgDP (condensed from the kit insert)

Components in each 192-test fibrinostika FgDP kit

1. Microelisa strips (murine monoclonal); two stripholders. Eight strips per holder, each containing 12 anti-FgDP/FbDP-coated wells; contained in a foil pack with silica gel desiccant.
2. Conjugate (murine monoclonal); four vials (lyophilized). HRP-labelled anti-FgDP.
3. Calibrator 900 (human); four vials (lyophilized). Plasma containing FgDP. Concentration after reconstitution 900 ng FE/ml.

Table 24.2 EIAs for degradation products of fibrinogen and fibrin

EIA specific for	Specificity of		Remarks
	Capture antibody	Tagging antibody	
Fibrinogen degradation products (FgDP)	Altered conformation in fibrin(ogen) degradation products (MoAb FDP-14)	Amino terminus of Aα-chains including FpA (MoAb Y 18)	Commercially available[a]. Duration of assay only 45 min. Uses dried MoAb precoated plates
D-dimer	Crosslinks in D-dimer	Panspecific anti-D MoAb	Commercially available[b]
D-dimer	Mainly for D-dimer	Panspecific antibody	Commercially available[c]
Fibrin degradation products (FbDP)	Altered conformation in fibrin(ogen) degradation products (MoAb FDP-14)	D-domain of both crosslinked and non-crosslinked FbDP (MoAb DD 13)	Commercially available[d]. Duration of assay only 45 min. Uses dried MoAb precoated plates
Total of degradation products (TDP) of fibrin (FbDP) plus those of fibrinogen (FgDP)	Altered conformation in fibrin(ogen) degradation products (MoAb FDP-14)	Mixture of two MoAbs (MoAb Y 18 and MoAb DD 13), see above	Commercially available[e]. Duration of assay only 45 min. Uses dried MoAb precoated plates

[a,d,e] From Organon Teknika, Veedijk 58, 2300 Turnhout, Belgium
[b] From MabCo, PO Box 475, Springwood Qld 4127, Australia; and American Diagnostica Inc., 222 Railroad Ave, PO Box 11625 Greenwich CT 06836-1165, USA
[c] From Diagnostica Stago, Asnières, France; and Boehringer Mannheim, Mannheim, Germany

196

4. Phosphate buffer concentrate; one bottle (100 ml). Dilute 25-fold before use.
5. TMB solution; one vial (2 ml). Tetramethylbenzidine in dimethyl-sulphoxide.
6. Substrate buffer; one vial (10 ml).
7. Urea peroxide; one tablet (140 mg).
8. Clamp and rod; one each. Closure for foil pack.
9. Plate sealers; six sheets. Perforated adhesive.

Storage instructions

1. Store all components at 2–8 °C when not in use. The expiration date printed on the kit indicates limits of stability.

2. The foil packs should be brought to room temperature (20–25 °C) before opening to prevent condensation on the microelisa strips. After the airtight foil pack has been opened, the strips are stable for 8 weeks at 2–8 °C, if the foil pack is resealed with the clamp and rod provided. The silica gel bag should not be removed.

Chemical or physical indications of instability

Alterations in the physical appearance of test kit material may indicate instability or deterioration. Expiration dates shown on component labels indicate the limits of stability.

Instruments

Any microelisa reader capable of transmitting a light source of 450 nm through a microelisa well may be used.

The aspiration/wash system must be capable of containing aspirated waste in a closed system and capable of dispensing a 300 μl volume. The manual provided by the instrument manufacturer should be reviewed for additional information regarding the following: (a) installation and special requirement; (b) operation principles, instructions, precautions, and hazards; (c) manufacturer's specifications and performance capabilities; (d) service and maintenance information.

Specimen collection and preparation

1. No special preparation of the patient is necessary, nor is fasting required.
2. Plasma samples (derived from citrate, heparin, oxalate or EDTA blood) must be used.
3. Specimens which have been repeatedly frozen and thawed, or those containing particulate matter, may give erroneous results.
4. Routinely, specimens should be diluted 20-fold in diluted phosphate buffer. If required, higher or lower dilutions of the specimens in diluted phosphate buffer may be used, but specimens must be diluted at least 10-fold.

(The kit inserts of all three EIAs state that the test samples should be diluted at least 10-fold (the routine dilution is 20-fold). On the basis of our recent experience we know that lower dilution factors are permitted. The lower detection limit of the assay is between 33 and 11 ng/ml.)

5. Specimens should be free of microbial contamination and may be stored at 2–8 °C for 1 week. Fresh specimens may be stored for 1 year at −20 °C (or lower).

6. For special applications when prolonged stability is required (e.g. samples taken after thrombolytic treatment), aprotinin at a final concentration of 100 ki.u./ml and heparin at a final concentration of 50 i.u./ml may be added to the samples.

Reagent preparation

Reagents and samples should be at room temperature (20–25 °C) before beginning the test, and can remain at room temperature during testing. Return reagents to 2–8 °C after use. All vessels used for preparation of reagents must be cleaned thoroughly and rinsed finally with distilled water. A clean disposable container must be used for each preparation of substrate.

Phosphate buffer

1. Check phosphate buffer concentrate for salt crystal formation. If crystals have formed in the solution, resolubilize concentrate by warming at 37 °C until crystals dissolve.

2. Dilute the phosphate buffer concentrate 1:25 with distilled water. Prepare at least 100 ml of diluted buffer for each microelisa strip used.

3. Add 2 weeks to the date of preparation and record on the container label.

Peroxide/substrate buffer

1. Dissolve the urea peroxide tablet in 10 ml distilled water and mix. The solution will contain some insoluble material, but this does not affect test results; therefore, filtration is not necessary.

2. Pipette 1.0 ml of the urea peroxide solution into the substrate buffer.

3. Relabel vial 'peroxide/substrate buffer'. Peroxide/substrate buffer is stable for 1 year if stored at 2–8 °C in the dark. The remaining urea peroxide solution may be discarded.

Conjugate. Pipette 6.0 ml diluted phosphate buffer into the vial. One vial is sufficient for four strips. Shake the vial gently and leave for at least 15 min before use. Reconstituted conjugate is stable for 4 weeks if stored at 2–8 °C.

Calibrator 900. Pipette 1.5 ml diluted phosphate buffer into the vial. One vial is sufficient for four strips. Shake the vial gently and leave for at least 15 min before use. Reconstituted calibrator 900 (concentration 900 ng FE/ml) is stable for 4 weeks if stored at 2–8 °C. Diluted calibrators are not stable; therefore, dilute calibrator 900 only for immediate use.

TMB solution.   The TMB solution contains dimethyl sulphoxide, an irritant to skin and mucous membranes. It should be protected from excessive exposure to light. TMB solution is used to prepare TMB substrate which is not stable; therefore, prepare only the amount needed for immediate use. Note: Solutions containing TMB should not come into contact with metal or metal ions since this may give rise to unwanted colour formation.

Procedural notes and precautions

Microelisa strips, conjugate, and calibrator 900 used in an assay must be of the same master lot number. Materials should not be used after the expiration date shown on the package label. Components and test specimens should be at room temperature (20–25 °C) before testing begins. Return the reagents to 2–8 °C after use.

Strips of the microelisa plate are removable. Store unused strips as described in 'Storage instructions'. Before testing begins, the user should inspect the microelisa strip-holder and ensure that all wells are secure. Strip-holders should be handled with care to ensure that no strip is dislodged during testing.

1. Microelisa strips may be used only once.
2. Ensure that the microelisa strips are well sealed during incubations.
3. To avoid contamination, do not touch the top of the strips or the edge of the wells with fingers or pipette tips, especially when pipetting samples, calibrators or conjugate.
4. All pipetting steps should be performed with the utmost care and accuracy. A separate disposable tip should be used for each sample, to avoid cross-contamination. Avoid microbial or any other contamination of reagents by using aseptic technique to remove aliquots from original vials.
5. The test samples, calibrators and conjugate must be well mixed before use.
6. Remove any bubbles in the well by gentle tapping.
7. If the well cannot be filled with conjugate or substrate immediately after washing, the strips may be placed upside-down on a wet absorbent tissue for no longer than 15 min.
8. If a water bath is used for incubation of the microelisa strip-holder, ensure that the bottom of all wells is in contact with the water.
9. If an incubator is used for 37 °C incubation of the microelisa strips, refrain from opening the door during the incubation time. Heat transfer in an incubator is enhanced by the presence of high humidity. This can be achieved by placing a tray of water or water-saturated paper towelling in the incubator.

Wash procedure

1. Incomplete washing will adversely affect the test outcome.
2. The wash procedure consists of an initial aspiration of well contents followed by filling the wells (approximately 0.3 ml) with diluted phosphate buffer. This should be done four times.
3. After the last aspiration, the wash procedure is completed by drying the top of the microelisa strips and strip-holder by blotting with absorbent tissue to prevent cross-contamination of wells.
4. Vacuum aspirate the well contents and wash buffer into a waste flask.
5. Routine maintenance of aspiration/wash system is strongly recommended to prevent carry-over from specimens containing a high concentration.
6. The aspiration/wash system should be flushed with copious amounts of water upon completion of the final wash of the assay.

Test procedure

Note: In each test run a maximum of four strips must be assayed.

1. Prepare serial 3-fold dilutions (3-, 9-, 27- and 81-fold) of an aliquot of calibrator 900 with diluted phosphate buffer (e.g. 150 μl with 300 μl buffer and homogenize; 150 μl of this 3-fold dilution with 300 μl buffer and homogenize, etc.). Calibrator 300, calibrator 100, calibrator 33, and calibrator 11 are now ready for use.
2. Fit the strip-holder with the required number of microelisa strips. If the microelisa washer used requires a full plate, use uncoated strips to complete the strip-holder.
3. The negative control (diluted phosphate buffer), calibrators and test samples are first pipetted into uncoated wells of polystyrene plates. The 20-fold dilution of test samples can be performed in the wells (e.g. 10 μl sample with 190 μl diluted phosphate buffer and homogenize). Distribution may be as follows:

If one strip is used:

Negative control	in A1
Calibrator 11	in A2
Calibrator 33	in A3
Calibrator 100	in A4
Calibrator 300	in A5
Calibrator 900	in A6

Test samples in the next wells.

If two or more strips are used and samples are in duplicate:

Negative control	in A1,B1
Calibrator 11	in A2,B2
Calibrator 33	in A3,B3
Calibrator 100	in A4,B4

Calibrator 300   in A5,B5
Calibrator 900   in A6,B6
Test samples in the next wells.

After filling, transfer with a 12-channel pipette 100 µl of each well to the corresponding well of the microelisa strips.

4. Cover the strips with adhesive plate sealer and incubate at 37 °C for 15 min.
5. Wash each well four times with diluted phosphate buffer (refer to 'Wash procedure').
6. Pipette 100 µl conjugate into each well.
7. Cover the strips with a new plate sealer and incubate at 37 °C for 15 min.
8. Wash each well four times with diluted phosphate buffer.
9. During incubation, prepare TMB substrate. Allow TMB solution to reach room temperature (20–25 °C) and check that the TMB is completely melted (melting point 18 °C). The TMB substrate for four strips is prepared as follows: Pipette 0.5 ml peroxide/substrate buffer into 5.0 ml distilled water contained in a new disposable vial and mix. Add 100 µl TMB solution and mix. The TMB substrate must be almost colourless when used.
10. Pipette 100 µl TMB substrate into each well.
11. Incubate at 37 °C for 10 min. Strips should not be covered with a plate sealer.
12. Stop the reaction by pipetting 100 µl of 1 mol/L (2 N) sulphuric acid into each well (maintain the same sequence and time intervals used for TMB substrate addition). Plates should be read within 1 h.
13. Blank the microelisa reader on air (without strip-holder and strips) and read the absorbance of the solution in each well at 450 nm.

Calculation of the test results

Calculations should be made separately for each stripholder.

Qualification of negative control (NC) and calibrator (CA$_i$) values.   Eliminate any individual NC ≥ 0.250. Eliminate any individual CA$_i$ outside the instrument's linear measuring range. Eliminate any individual CA$_i$ preventing a monotonous increase of the mean calibrator (CA$_i$X) values by their rank.

Test validity.   A test run is valid if at least one negative control remains; not more than one CA$_i$ has been eliminated; CA900X ≥ 1.000 and (CA900X − CA100X) > (CA100X − CA11X).

Quantitative determination.   Plot the CA$_i$X values on semi-logarithmic paper. Draw straight lines through the points. Read the sample concentration from this broken line. Multiply with the dilution factor (usually 20) to obtain the FgDP concentration in the original sample.

Remark: If needed for evaluation samples with absorbances exceeding the instrument's linear measuring range should be retested in a higher dilution.

Sample calculations

Absorbance

NC = 0.027;	0.031	NCX = 0.029
CA11 = 0.048;	0.056	CA11X = 0.052
CA33 = 0.128;	0.154	CA33X = 0.141
CA100 = 0.367;	0.397	CA100X = 0.382
CA300 = 0.982;	1.028	CA300X = 1.005
CA900 = 1.699;	1.797	CA900X = 1.748

Acceptance criteria

Eliminate any $NC \geq 0.250$
  None eliminated

Eliminate any CA_i outside the instrument's linear measuring range
  None eliminated

Eliminate any CA_i preventing

$$CA900X > CA300X > CA100X > CA33X > CA11X$$

  None eliminated

Ensure that the following is within specified acceptance criteria:

At least one NC remains	Pass
Not more than one CA_i has been eliminated	Pass
$CA900X \geq 1.000$ and	Pass
$(CA900X - CA100X) > (CA100X - CA11X)$ $1.366 > 0.330$	Pass

References

1. Doolittle RF. Fibrinogen and fibrin. Sci Am 1981; 245: 92–101.
2. Graeff H, Hafter R. Detection and relevance of cross-linked fibrin derivatives in blood. Semin Thromb Haemostas 1982; 8: 57–68.
3. Gaffney PJ, Perry MJ. 'Giant' fibrin fragments and thrombosis. Thromb Haemostas 1985; 54: 931 (abstract).
4. Gaffney PJ, Creighton LC, Harris R, Perry MJ. Monoclonal antibodies (MABS) to crosslinked fibrin fragments. Their characterization and potential clinical use. In: Müller-Berghaus G. *et al.*, eds. Fibrinogen and its derivatives: biochemistry, physiology and pathophysiology. Amsterdam: Excerpta Medica, 1986; 273–84.
5. Merskey C, Lalezazi P, Johnson AJ. A rapid simple sensitive method for measuring fibrinolytic split products in human serum. Proc Soc Exp Biol Med NY 1969; 131: 871–5.
6. Connaghan DG, Francis DW, Ryan DH, Marder VJ. Prevalence and clinical implications of heparin-associated false positive tests for serum fibrin(ogen) degradation products. Am J Clin Pathol 1986; 86: 304–10.
7. Haverkate F, Timan G, Nieuwenhuizen W. Anticlotting properties of fragments D from human fibrinogen and fibrin. Eur J Clin Invest 1979; 9: 253–5.

8. Nieuwenhuizen W, Gravesen M. Anticoagulant and calcium-binding properties of high molecular weight derivatives of human fibrinogen, produced by plasmin (fragments X). Biochim Biophys Acta 1981; 668: 81–8.
9. Nieuwenhuizen W, Voskuilen M, Hermans J. Anticoagulant and calcium-binding properties of high molecular weight derivatives of human fibrinogen (plasmin fragments Y). Biochim Biophys Acta 1982; 708: 313–16.
10. Koopman J, Haverkate F, Koppert PW, Nieuwenhuizen W, Brommer EJP, van der Werf WGC. New enzyme immunoassay of fibrin–fibrinogen degradation products in plasma using a monoclonal antibody. J Lab Clin Med 1987; 109: 75–84.
11. Marder VJ, Shulman NR. High molecular weight derivatives of human fibrinogen produced by plasmin II. Mechanism of their anticoagulant activity. J Biol Chem 1969; 244: 2120–4.
12. Gaffney PJ, Perry MJ. Unreliability of current serum fibrin degradation products (FDP) assays. Thromb Haemostas 1985; 53: 301–2.
13. Niewiarowski S, Stewart GJ, Marder VJ. Formation of highly ordered polymers fibrinogen and fibrin degradation products. Biochim Biophys Acta 1970; 221: 326–41.
14. Koppert PW, Koopman J, Haverkate F, Nieuwenhuizen W. Production and characterization of a monoclonal antibody reactive with a specific neoantigenic determinant (comprising Bβ 54-118) in degradation products of fibrin and of fibrinogen. Blood 1986; 68: 437–41.
15. Koppert PW, Huijsmans CMG, Nieuwenhuizen W. A monoclonal antibody, specific for human fibrinogen, fibrinopeptide A-containing fragments and not reacting with free fibrinopeptide A. Blood 1985; 66: 503–7.
16. Koppert PW, Kuipers W, Hoegee-de Nobel E, Brommer EJP, Koopman J, Nieuwenhuizen W. A quantitative enzyme immunoassay for primary fibrinogenolysis products in plasma. Thromb Haemostas 1987; 57: 25–8.
17. Koppert PW, Hoegee-de Nobel E, Nieuwenhuizen W. A monoclonal antibody-based enzyme immunoassay for fibrin degradation products in plasma. Thromb Haemostas 1988; 59: 310–15.
18. Kroneman H, Nieuwenhuizen W, Knot EAR. Monoclonal antibody-based plasma assays for fibrin(ogen) and derivatives, and their clinical relevance. Blood Coagul Fibrinol 1990; 1: 91–111.
19. Scheefers-Borchel U, Müller-Berghaus G, Fuhge P, Eberle R, Heimburger N. Discrimination between fibrin and fibrinogen by a monoclonal antibody against a synthetic peptide. Proc Natl Acad Sci USA 1985; 82: 7091–5.
20. Müller-Berghaus G, Scheefers-Borchel U, Fuhge P, Eberle R, Heimburger N. Detection of fibrin in plasma by a monoclonal antibody against the aminoterminus of the alpha-chain of fibrin. Scand J Lab Invest 1985; 45: 145–51.
21. Scheefers-Borchel U, Müller-Berghaus G, Fuhge P, Heimburger N. Discrimination between fibrin and fibrinogen by a monoclonal antibody against a synthetic hexapeptide representing the amino-terminus of the alpha-chain of fibrin. In: Lane DA, ed. Fibrinogen, fibrin formation and fibrinolysis. Berlin: Walter de Gruyter 1986; 253–60.

25
Bβ 15–42 peptide

A. HAEBERLI

INTRODUCTION

Thrombin is a key serine protease of the coagulation cascade. It attacks fibrinogen by first cleaving off two fibrinopeptide A molecules from the N-terminal part of the Aα-chain, thus converting fibrinogen to fibrin I, then cleaving off two fibrinopeptide B molecules from the N-terminal part of the Bβ-chain, thus transforming fibrin I to fibrin II, mostly just called fibrin (see Chapter 24).

Plasmin, on the other hand, is the key enzyme of the fibrinolytic system. The major substrate for plasmin is fibrin, although in certain circumstances also fibrinogen is degraded (fibrinogenolysis). During fibrinolysis one of the first attacks of plasmin is directed towards the C-terminal part of the Aα-chain, whereby a large peptide with a molecular weight of about 48 000 is cleaved off. A second highly susceptible cleavage site is located in the N-terminal part of the Bβ-chain, between Arg-42 and Ala-43[1]. If the substrate is fibrinogen, or in rare cases fibrin I, the Bβ 1–42 peptide is released by the action of plasmin, or, in the more frequent case, where fibrin is the substrate, the Bβ 15–42* peptide is formed, since the first 14 amino acids of the N-terminal part of the Bβ-chain have been cleaved off by thrombin as fibrinopeptide B.

Several assay systems for the evaluation of the fibrinolytic activity by the measurement of the products of degradation of fibrin(ogen) have been developed. The focus of most of these assays was directed towards the determination of the high molecular weight fragments such as D-dimer stemming from crosslinked fibrin and other fibrin degradation products. For

---

* The correct nomenclature for this peptide would be β 15–42, since it is a degradation product of fibrin. Since Bβ 15–42 has been generally used for this peptide by most authors it will be used throughout this chapter.

the determination of smaller fragments the most prominent assays are radioimmunoassays or ELISAs for the peptides Bβ 15–42 and Bβ 1–42[2-4].

PATHOPHYSIOLOGY

In 1982 Kudryk et al. presented a radioimmunoassay (RIA) for the determination of the Bβ 15–42 peptide in plasma[2]. Since its introduction as a commercial kit by Imco (Stockholm, Sweden) this RIA has been used to document enhanced fibrinolytic activity in different diseases such as postoperative deep venous thrombosis in malignancy[5], in neoplasia[6], in glomerulonephritis[7] and in nephrotoxicity with rejection of renal transplants[8], in diabetes[9] and in liver cirrhosis[10]. Fibrinolytic therapy of deep venous thrombosis with urokinase[11] or with tissue plasminogen activator in acute myocardial infarction[12-14] was followed by the measurement of fibrinolytic degradation products such as the Bβ 15–42 peptide. The exercise-induced activation of fibrinolysis in coronary artery disease was evaluated by the determination of the Bβ 15–42 peptide[15].

The Bβ 15–42 RIA has also been used for in vitro studies, e.g. to follow the activation of plasminogen by urokinase in the presence of fibrin[16], and the effects of inhibitors such as α_2-antiplasmin[17] or tranexamic acid[18] on fibrinolytic or fibrinogenolytic activity.

METHOD OF ASSAY

Two assay methods for the measurement of the Bβ 15–42 peptide have been described and used so far. One is an ELISA developed by Kudryk and co-workers using a monoclonal antibody against the Bβ 15–42 peptide[3,19]. This assay was manufactured and supplied by the New York Blood Center until recently. Although crossreacting to some extent with the Bβ 1–42 peptide, it was much more susceptible to the Bβ 15–42 peptide, thus allowing the differentiation between fibrinolytic and fibrinogenolytic degradation products[20]. Unfortunately this assay is no longer commercially available; therefore it will not be discussed in detail here.

The other assay, also developed by Kudryk et al.[2], is a competitive radioimmunoassay (RIA) manufactured by Imco (Stockholm, Sweden). It is not a ready-to-use kit. Imco supplies only the antiserum, the Bβ 15–42 standard, lyophilized and undiluted, and the Bβ 15–42 peptide for radioiodination. All buffers, dilutions of antiserum and standards, as well as the radioiodination of the Bβ 15–42 peptide have to be performed in house. The assay performs well, but it is appropriate only for laboratories familiar with radioimmunoassays.

The RIA prepared by Imco as described here has two critical aspects. First, the antibody supplied by Imco against the Bβ 15–42 peptide also recognizes the Bβ 1–42 peptide (equimolar reaction). Therefore it is not possible to differentiate between fibrinolysis (Bβ 15–42 peptide) and fibrinogenolysis (Bβ 1–42 peptide). This differentiation, however, is of considerable importance in clinical situations, because it allows establishment of whether the degradation products are stemming from fibrin or from fibrinogen. Second, the antibody against the Bβ 15–42 peptide also reacts with intact fibrinogen. It is therefore essential to remove the plasma fibrinogen before the assay may be performed, in order to avoid falsely elevated values due to the binding of fibrinogen to the antibody.

Bβ 15–42 RADIOIMMUNOASSAY (Imco)

The Bβ 15–42 radioimmunoassay is a competitive binding assay. It is based on a competition between unlabelled Bβ 15–42 peptide and the ^{125}I-labelled Bβ 15–42 (=tracer) for the limited amount of antibody binding sites. As the concentration of unlabelled Bβ 15–42 peptide increases, less of the tracer will be bound to the antibody.

The standard curve is drawn by plotting the percentage of tracer bound in each standard versus its concentration on a semi-log or logit–log scale. The Bβ 15–42 concentration in the unknown sample is determined by comparison of the percentage labelled Bβ 15–42 bound to the standard curve.

As compared to the assay procedure suggested by Imco some modifications have been introduced in our laboratory, and used successfully for several years.

For reasons of clarity the whole RIA procedure will be described including the modifications mentioned below.

Modifications

As compared to the RIA assay protocol included with the reagents the following modifications have been introduced and used in our laboratory for several years.

1. The number of buffers has been reduced from six to four, without any change in quality of performance. For reasons of clarity the numerical order of the buffers has been kept identical to the one described by Imco.
2. An immobilized second antibody has been introduced.

An attempt to replace ethanol by bentonite for the removal of fibrinogen from plasma (as described in the FPA RIA procedure) was not successful.

1. *Reagents*

1.1. *Buffers* (numerical order identical to Imco)

Buffer I (used for iodination): 0.4 mol/L Na-phosphate, pH 7.4.

Buffer II (Tris-buffer): 0.05 mol/L Tris, 0.1 mol/L NaCl, 0.01 mol/L EDTA, adjusted to pH 7.4 with 5 mol/L HCl; 0.02% sodium azide.

Buffer III omitted.

Buffer IV (Tris-buffer supplemented with albumin): 20 KIE aprotinin and 1 mg bovine serum albumin (RIA grade) per ml are added to buffer II before use.

Buffer V omitted.

Buffer VI (Tris-buffer supplemented with ethanol): ethanol (95%) is added to buffer IV to make the final concentration 25% (volume/volume).

1.2. *Polyclonal anti Bβ 15–42 serum* (Imco): 0.5 ml/ampoule
The antiserum is prediluted 1:10 with buffer IV. This predilution is stored in 50–100 μl aliquots at −70 °C.

1.3. *Bβ 15–42 Standard* (Imco): 25 μg/ampoule
The standard is diluted to 80 nmol/L in the following way: The entire standard (25 μg) is first dissolved in 1 ml of water and the volume is adjusted to 10 ml with buffer IV: 2500 ng/ml. 1 ml aliquots are stored frozen at −70 °C until use. Second dilution: 1 ml of the standard solution containing 2500 ng/ml is further diluted to a final volume of 10.3 ml with buffer IV. This solution has a concentration of 80 nmol/L in respect to the Bβ 15–42 peptide. It is stored in 0.5 ml aliquots at −70 °C (compare section 3.1).

1.4. *Bβ 15–42 peptide for radioiodination* (Imco): 50 μg/ampoule
The peptide is dissolved in 125 μl of buffer I. Aliquots of 25 μl are kept frozen at −70 °C until used for iodination.

1.5. *Anticoagulant for blood collection*
Heparin–aprotinin anticoagulant: 0.5 ml containing 500 KIE aprotinin and 500 IU heparin dissolved in physiologic saline for 4.5 ml whole blood.

1.6. *Immobilized second antibody*
For the precipitation of the antigen–antibody complexes an immobilized second antibody, e.g. immunobead second antibody, goat–anti-rabbit IgG (BioRad Laboratories) is used. To one vial 50 ml of buffer II is added. The suspension is kept on a rotating table 30 min prior to use. The dissolved antibody suspension can be stored in the cold room at 4 °C for 3 weeks.

1.7. *Wash solution*
This solution is used to wash the centrifuged second antibody–first antibody complex. It is buffer IV with 0.1% Tween 20 added.

Plasma preparation

2.1. *Blood collection*
Blood should be taken from volunteers or patients only after a rest of at least 30 min, to avoid artificial activation of the fibrinolytic system due to physical exercise. The blood is collected into the recommended anticoagulants

by smooth aspiration under a stasis of not more than 50 mmHg. Vacutainer tubes should not be used, since they give rise to elevated values, for unknown reasons. The syringes should be well mixed immediately after the collection of blood and placed in an ice bath. Centrifugation must be carried out at 2000 g for 20 min at 4 °C. The plasma is then carefully removed and either processed according to section 2.3 or frozen at −70 °C.

2.2. Quality control plasma

Blood is collected from at least 10 healthy volunteers. All plasmas are pooled in equal volumes. The 0.5 ml aliquots are frozen at −70 °C until use. One aliquot is included in each RIA.

2.3. Removal of fibrinogen

Ethanol (95%) must be precooled at 0 °C for at least 1 h before use; 0.5 ml of anticoagulated plasma is mixed with 0.5 ml of ice-cold ethanol (95%). The mixtures are allowed to stand for 30 min in an ice bath. The tubes are then centrifuged at 2000 g at 4 °C for 20 min. The supernatant is transferred to another tube and kept in the ice bath for an additional 30 min. The centrifugation is repeated at the same conditions as the first time. The top ($\approx 300 \mu l$) of the supernatant is removed; 150 μl of the supernatant are used for the predilution step prior to the RIA (see section 3.2). The rest of the supernatant has to be discarded, because storing and reuse of the supernatant may give rise to erroneous values.

3. RIA procedure

3.1. Standard dilution

The standard solution containing 80 nmol/L (see section 1.3) is diluted 1:10 with buffer VI. The new concentration is 8 nmol/L. This is the highest standard in the RIA. A serial standard dilution starting with 8 nmol/L is made by 1:1 dilution in buffer VI. Thus the following standard concentrations will be obtained and used in the RIA: 8 nmol/L, 4 nmol/L, 2 nmol/L, 1 nmol/L, 0.5 nmol/L, 0.25 nmol/L, 0.125 nmol/L and 0.063 nmol/L.

3.2. Dilution of the plasma supernatant

In order to reduce the ethanol concentration from 50% to 25% in the RIA tubes, the plasma supernatants (after ethanol precipitation) have to be diluted before adding them to the RIA tubes: 150 μl of the plasma supernatant (see section 2.3) is mixed with 150 μl of buffer IV (buffer *not* containing ethanol). After this dilution the plasma supernatants can be introduced into the RIA.

3.3. Antiserum dilution

The final dilution of the antiserum may be 1:1500 to 1:4000, depending on the lot of antiserum. B_0 should be between 30% and 50%. The final dilution from the prediluted antiserum aliquots (see section 1.2) is made with buffer IV.

3.4. *Tracer dilution*
The radiolabelled Bβ 1,5–42 peptide is diluted with buffer so that 50 μl contain approximately 20 000 cpm.

3.5. *Assay*
Aliquots are added in the following order according to the protocol:

First day
  buffer VI for total counts, NSB and B_0
  standard dilution in buffer VI
  plasma sample supernatants, prediluted (see section 3.2)
  tracer diluted in buffer IV
  incubation for 15–30 min at room temperature
  antiserum diluted in buffer IV to the working dilution
  mixing and incubation for 16–18 h at 4 °C

Protocol (see Table 25.1)

Table 25.1   Protocol

Tube no.	Sample	Buffer VI (μl)	Standard or sample (μl)	Antiserum (μl)	Tracer (μl)
1–3	Total counts	200	–	–	50
4–6	NSB	200	–	–	50
7–9	B_0	100	–	100	50
10–12	Standard 8 nmol/L	–	100	100	50
13–15	Standard 4	–	100	100	50
16–18	Standard 2	–	100	100	50
19–21	Standard 1	–	100	100	50
22–24	Standard 0.5	–	100	100	50
25–27	Standard 0.25	–	100	100	50
28–30	Standard 0.125	–	100	100	50
31–33	Standard 0.063	–	100	100	50
34–35	Sample 1	–	100	100	50
36–37	Sample 2				
38–39	...				

Second day
  suspend immobilized second antibody (e.g. immunobead second antibody, BioRad Laboratories) and add 300 μl to each tube except to tube 1–3 (total counts)
  incubate at 4 °C for 1 h on a rotating table
  centrifuge at 2000 g for 10 min at 4 °C
  discard supernatant
  wash with 1 ml of wash solution (compare section 1.7)
  centrifuge at 2000 g for 10 min at 4 °C
  discard supernatant
  repeat washing procedure
  count precipitate for radioactivity

the concentration of the Bβ 15–42 peptide in the samples is determined by reading the percentage of bound tracer on the standard curve either on a semi-log or on a logit–log scale

The dilution of the plasma samples due to the ethanol precipitation and the dilution of the ethanol supernatant to decrease the ethanol concentration to 25% has to be considered in the calculation of the final concentration of the peptide.

Iodination of the Bβ 15–42 peptide

The iodination of the peptide is carried out exactly as described in the instructions given by Imco.

NORMAL VALUES

Each laboratory has to establish its own normal values, since the blood collection and the processing of the plasma (alcohol precipitation) has a considerable effect on the Bβ 15–42 values. In our laboratory (using the conditions as described) normal values are 0.92 ± 0.5 nmol/L ($n = 31$) with a range of 0.15–2.9 nmol/L.

The recovery of the Bβ 15–42 peptide after the ethanol precipitation of the plasma is 85–95%. The normal values given here have not been corrected for this recovery.

Quite large variations of normal values have been described by other laboratories with values such as 0.4 nmol/L[2], 1.9 nmol/L[15], 2.2 nmol/L[7], 4 nmol/L[10], and even 10 nmol/L[6].

These variations may certainly be partially due to blood sampling and blood processing problems. In addition, elevated values can easily be observed in healthy persons as well as in patients after physical exercise. This means that persons have to rest at least 30 minutes before blood is collected.

PERSPECTIVES

The results obtained with the Bβ 15–42 RIA should be interpreted with caution. Falsely elevated values may easily be obtained due to problems during blood sampling, blood processing or improper removal of fibrinogen. Moreover, since the antibody binds the Bβ 15–42 and the Bβ 1–42 in a equimolar ratio, the assay does not allow differentiation between fibrinolysis and fibrinogenolysis.

Other new assays using monoclonal antibodies specific for fibrin or fibrinogen degradation products are certainly more selective for the documentation of fibrinolysis, since they differentiate more clearly between fibrinolysis and fibrinogenolysis (see Chapter 24).

References

1. Takagi T, Doolittle RF. Amino acid sequence studies on plasmin-derived fragments of human fibrinogen: amino-terminal sequence of intermediate and terminal fragments. Biochemistry 1975; 14: 940–6.
2. Kudryk B, Robinson D, Netré C, Hessel B, Blombäck M, Blombäck B. Measurement in human blood of fibrinogen/fibrin fragments containing the Bβ 15–42 sequence. Thromb Res 1982; 25: 277–91.
3. Kudryk B, Rohoza A, Ahadi M, Chin J, Wiebe ME. A monoclonal antibody with ability to distinguish between NH$_2$-terminal fragments derived from fibrinogen and fibrin. Mol Immunol 1983; 20: 1191–200.
4. Weitz JI, Koehn JA, Canfield RE, Landman SL, Friedman R. Development of a radioimmunoassay for the fibrinogen-derived peptide Bβ 1–42. Blood 1986; 67: 1014–22.
5. Douglas JT, Blamey SL, Lowe, GDO, Carter DC, Forbes CD. Plasma beta-thromboglobulin, fibrinopeptide A and Bβ 15–42 antigen in relation to postoperative DVT, malignancy and stanozolol treatment. Thromb Haemostas 1985; 53: 235–8.
6. Fareed J, Bick RL, Squillaci G, Walenga JM, Bermes EW. Molecular markers of hemostatic disorders: Implications in the diagnosis and therapeutic management of thrombotic and bleeding disorders. Clin Chem 1983; 29: 1641–58.
7. Tomura S, Oono Y, Kuriyama R, Takeuchi J. Plasma concentrations of fibrinpeptide A and fibrinopeptide Bβ 15–42 in glomerulonephritis and the nephrotic syndrome. Arch Intern Med 1985; 145: 1033–5.
8. Morozumi K, Kano T, Kobayashi M, Shinmura I, Yoshida A, Fujinami T, Otaguro K, Uchida K, Yamada N, Tominaga Y, Takagi H. The clinical significance of urinary fibrinopeptide A and fibrinopeptide Bβ 15–42 in chronic rejection and nephrotoxicity of renal allograft recipients immunosuppressed with cyclosporin. Transpl Proc 1987; 19: 1791–4.
9. Marongiu F, Conti M, Mameli G, Sorano GG, Cossu E, Cirillo R, Balestrieri A. Is the imbalance between thrombin and plasmin activity in diabetes related to the behaviour of antiplasmin activity? Thromb Res 1990; 58: 91–9.
10. Marongiu F, Mameli G, Acca MR, Mulas G, Medda A, Tronci MB, Mamusa AM, Balestrieri A. Fibrinopeptide A and Bβ 15–42 in liver cirrhosis. Haemostasis 1988; 18: 126–8.
11. Urano T, Kamiya T, Sakaguchi S, Takada Y, Takada, A. Fibrinogenolysis and fibrinolysis in normal volunteers and patients with thrombosis after infusion of urokinase. Thromb Res 1985; 39: 145–55.
12. Owen J, Friedman KD, Grossman BA, Wilkins C, Berke AD, Powers ER. Quantitation of fragment X formation during thrombolytic therapy with streptokinase and tissue plasminogen activator. J Clin Invest 1987; 79: 1642–7.
13. Eisenberg PR, Sobel BE, Jaffe AS. Characterization in vivo of the fibrin specificity of activators of the fibrinolytic system. Circulation 1988; 78: 592–7.
14. Ring ME, Butman SM, Bruck DC, Feinberg WM, Corrigan JJ. Fibrin metabolism in patients with acute myocardial infarction during and after treatment with tissue-type plasminogen activator. Thromb Haemostas 1988; 60: 428–33.
15. Small M, Simpson I, McGhie I, Douglas JT, Lowe GDO, Forbes CD. The effect of exercise on thrombin and plasmin generation in middle-aged men. Haemostasis 1987; 17: 371–6.
16. Urano T, Takada Y, Takada A. The enhanced activation of Glu-plasminogen by urokinase in the presence of fibrin or des A-fibrin as measured by the release of Bβ peptide and FDP. Thromb Res 1984; 36: 429–35.
17. Takada A, Makino Y, Takada Y. Release of Bβ peptides from fibrinogen or fibrin in the presence of α_2-antiplasmin. Thromb Res 1986; 42: 1–9.
18. Takada A, Makino Y, Takada Y. Effects of tranexamic acid on fibrinolysis, fibrinogenolysis and amidolysis. Thromb Res 1986; 42: 39–47.
19. Kudryk B, Rohoza A, Ahadi M, Chin J, Wiebe ME. Specificity of a monoclonal antibody for the NH$_2$-terminal region of fibrin. Mol Immunol 1984; 21: 89–94.
20. Lawler CM, Bovill EG, Stump DC, Collen DJ, Mann KG, Tracy RP. Fibrin fragment D-dimer and fibrinogen Bβ peptides in plasma as markers of clot lysis during thrombolytic therapy in acute myocardial infarction. Blood 1990; 76: 1341–8.

26
The venous occlusion test in fibrinolysis assays

J. JESPERSEN

INTRODUCTION

Since its introduction more than 30 years ago[1,2], the venous occlusion test (VO-test) has been widely used to assess the systemic fibrinolytic capacity after venous occlusion. In the mid-eighties the VO-test was included in the ECAT procedures and in the ECAT clinical trials, e.g. the Angina Pectoris Study.

Pathophysiology

In a number of cross-sectional or case–control studies a poor fibrinolytic response after venous occlusion has frequently been observed in patients with recurrent venous thrombosis[3–6]. At least five families have been identified with recurrent venous thrombosis and an impaired fibrinolytic response to venous occlusion[7–11]. The incidence of abnormal fibrinolysis in patients with venous thrombosis is about 30%[4,6,12], and the VO-test result appears also to have a predictive value for the recurrence of venous thrombosis[13].

A reduced fibrinolytic response after the VO-test characterizes patients with ischaemic heart disease, as revealed from case–control studies[14–17]. Decreased fibrinolytic capacity after venous occlusion has recently been shown to have a predictive value as a risk marker for reinfarction and cardiac death among young survivors of acute myocardial infarction[18].

Assessment of the fibrinolytic capacity following VO-test is often performed by a global screening test – based for instance on the determination of the fibrinolytic activity in plasma euglobulin fractions. Results of such global assays were thought to reflect mainly the systemic t-PA activity. However, significant contributions of both the factor XII-dependent pathway and the pro-urokinase/urokinase have been observed, probably through the generation of plasmin via the t-PA system and subsequent activation of the intrinsic system[19-24]. The results might also be seriously affected by the presence of inhibitors[24].

The introduction of more specific assays has made it possible to determine t-PA[25,26] and PAI-1[27-30] activity and protein concentration[31]. By means of these techniques an impaired response following the VO-test has been attributed to either an increased baseline level of plasminogen activator inhibitors or to a deficient release of t-PA from the vessel wall[4-6,32,33].

PRINCIPLE OF THE TEST

When external pressure is applied to the arm by a blood cuff several factors cause a rise in the fibrinolytic activity, e.g. accumulation, extravasation of fluid, clearance, and metabolic changes. Although Keber[34] provided strong evidence that during venous occlusion the accumulation of t-PA can be explained merely by continuously produced t-PA of the endothelium and change of clearance via the liver, an acute release of t-PA cannot be excluded[35].

EQUIPMENT

1. Blood pressure cuff, balloon and sphygmomanometer.
2. At least two blood test tubes placed in an ice-water bath (see Chapter 2 for details).

PERFORMING THE VO-TEST

1. The participant is asked to sit down in an easy chair or to lay down on a bed for at least 15 min.
2. From one arm blood is collected by venepuncture.
3. The blood pressure cuff is then wrapped around the other arm just above the elbow.
4. The cuff is inflated to a pressure 10–15 mmHg above diastolic pressure, i.e. the diastolic pressure is read from the manometer at the point where during gradual inflation Korotkov sounds disappear.
5. By squeezing the balloon now and then the pressure is maintained for 10 min.
6. Exactly 10 min after the inflation of the cuff to the desired level, venepuncture is performed in the congested arm vein.
7. Just before withdrawing the needle, the cuff should be deflated.

During the procedure the colour of the forearm skin turns purple and lighter patches may become visible. In the first few minutes some aching and tingling may be felt.

COMMENTS

To date the distinction between good and bad responders to the VO-test and the determination of global fibrinolytic activity or specific determination of components within the t-PA/PAI system have revealed wide interlaboratory variations[31]. Furthermore, no agreement exists about the required stimulation procedure, type of assays, degree of deviation from normal range, and whether correction for haemoconcentration is needed or not. Clearly the diversity of fibrinolytic assays and lack of standardization of the VO-test explain that so far there has been little practical, clinical impact. Thus, until a consensus is established on how to perform the VO-test and which assays to use its main application is in well-defined clinical trials. The choice at the introduction of the VO-test in the ECAT studies, of a venous occlusion duration of 10 min, was a compromise of the traditional 20 min[1,2] in order to avoid any severe complaints from the patients. Later, fortunately, the clinical value of 10 min venous occlusion was documented in a prospective study of patients with ischaemic heart disease[18]. With respect to which assays should be used, it is rcommended to assess the fibrinolytic activity by a global test followed by assessment of the individual components of the t-PA/PAI system involved[31]. However, this *Assay Procedure* manual might be an important platform in the needed standardization process. In the meantime each laboratory has had to describe any deviation from the suggested standardized procedure and establish its own reference material. Examples of such procedures are available (e.g. refs 4, 6, 12, 32, 35, 37, 38).

References

1. Nilsson IM, Robertson B. Effect of venous occlusion on coagulation and fibrinolytic components in normal subjects. Thromb Diath Haemorrh, 1968; 20: 397–408.
2. Robertson BR, Pandolfi M, Nilsson IM. 'Fibrinolytic capacity' in healthy volunteers as estimated from effect of venous occlusion of arms. Acta Chir Scand 1972; 138: 429–36.
3. Isacson S, Nilsson IM. Defective fibrinolysis in blood and vein walls in recurrent 'idiopathic' venous thrombosis. Acta Chir Scand 1972; 138: 313–9.
4. Nilsson IM, Ljungnér H, Tengborn L. Two different mechanisms in patients with venous thrombosis and defective fibrinolysis: low concentration of plasminogen activator or increased concentration of plasminogen activator inhibitor. Br Med J 1985; 290: 1453–6.
5. Stalder M, Hauert J, Kruithof EKO, Bachmann F. Release of vascular plasminogen activator (v-PA) after venous stasis: electrophoretic-zymographic analysis of free and complexed v-PA. Br J Haematol 1985; 61: 169–76.
6. Juhan-Vague I, Valadier J, Alessi MC, et al. Deficient t-PA release and elevated PA inhibitor levels in patients with spontaneous or recurrent deep venous thrombosis. Thromb Haemost. 1987; 57: 62–72.
7. Johansson L, Hedner U, Nilsson IM. A family with thromboembolic disease associated with deficient fibrinolytic activity in vessel wall. Acta Med Scand 1978; 203: 477–80.
8. Alexandre P, Larcan A, Briquel ME. Recurring thrombo-embolic accidents caused by family-related deficiency of the fibrinolysis system. Blut 1980; 41: 437–44.
9. Jorgensen M, Mortensen JZ, Madsen AG, Thorsen S, Jacobsen B. A family with reduced plasminogen activator activity in blood associated with recurrent venous thrombosis. Scand J Haematol 1982; 29: 217–23.
10. Stead NW, Bauer KA, Kinney TR, et al. Venous thrombosis in a family with defective release of vascular plasminogen activator and elevated plasma factor VIII/von Willebrand's factor. Am J Med 1983; 74: 33–9.
11. Boyko OB, Pizzo SV. Mesenteric vein thrombosis and vascular plasminogen activator. Arch Pathol Lab Med 1983; 107: 541–2.
12. Alessi MC, Juhan-Vague I, Valadier J, Philip-Joet C, Holvoet P, Collen D. Relevance of free tPA assay following venous occlusion in patients with venous thromboembolic disease. Thromb Haemost 1988; 59: 346–7.
13. Korninger C, Lechner K, Niessner H, Gössinger H, Kundi M. Impaired fibrinolytic capacity predisposes for recurrence of venous thrombosis. Thromb Haemost 1984; 52: 127–30.

14. Walker ID, Davidson JF, Hutton I, Lawrie TDV. Disordered 'fibrinolytic potential' in coronary heart disease. Thromb Res 1977; 10: 509–20.
15. Gritsyuk AI, Schogelsky VI. Evaluation of blood coagulation and prethrombotic state in patients with coronary atherosclerosis by application of controlled local venous blockade. Circulation 1979; 60: 220A.
16. Rawles JM, Warlow C, Ogston D. Fibrinolytic capacity of arm and leg veins after femoral shaft fracture and acute myocardial infarction. Br Med J 1975; 2: 61–2.
17. Hamsten A, Blombäck M, Wiman B, Svensson J, Szamosi A, de Faire U, Mettinger L. Haemostatic function in myocardial infarction. Br Heart J 1986; 55: 58–66.
18. Hamsten A, de Faire U, Walldius G et al. Plasminogen activator inhibitor in plasma: risk factor for recurrent myocardial infarction. Lancet 1987; 2: 3–9.
19. Jespersen J. The diurnal increase in euglobulin fibrinolytic activity in women using oral contraceptives and in normal women, and the generation of intrinsic fibrinolytic activity. Thromb Haemost 1986; 56: 183–8.
20. Rijken DC, Wijngaards G, Welbergen J. Relationship between tissue plasminogen activator and the activators in blood and vascular wall. Thromb Res 1980; 18: 815–30.
21. Kluft C, Wijngaards G, Jie AFH. The factor XII-independent plasminogen proactivator system of plasma includes urokinase-related activity. Thromb Haemost 1981; 46: 343.
22. Kluft C, Jie AFH. Interaction between the extrinsic and intrinsic system of fibrinolysis. In: Davidson JF et al, eds. Progress in clinical fibrinolysis and thrombolysis. Edinburgh: Churchill Livingstone 1979; 25–31.
23. Kluft C, Dooijewaard G, Emeis JJ. Role of the contact system in fibrinolysis. Semin Thromb Hemostas 1987; 13: 50–68.
24. Jespersen J. Pathophysiology and clinical aspects of fibrinolysis and inhibition of coagulation. Experimental and clinical studies with special reference to women on oral contraceptives and selected groups of thrombosis prone patients. Thesis. Dan Med Bull 1988; 35: 1–33.
25. Rijken DC, Juhan-Vague I, De Cock F, Collen D. Measurement of human tissue-type plasminogen activator by two-site immuno radiometric assay. J Lab Clin Med 1983; 101: 274–84.
26. Verheijen JH, Mullaart E, Chang GTG, Kluft C, Wijngaards G. A simple, sensitive spectrophotometric assay for extrinsic (tissue-type) plasminogen activator applicable to measurements in plasma. Thromb Haemost 1982; 48: 266–9.
27. Chmielewska J, Rånby M, Wiman B. Evidence for a rapid inhibitor to tissue plasminogen activator in plasma. Thromb Res 1983; 31: 427–36.
28. Kruithof EKO, Tran-Thang C, Ransijn A, Bachmann F. Demonstration of a fast-acting inhibitor of plasminogen activators in human plasma. Blood 1984; 64: 907–13.
29. Verheijen JH, Chang GTG, Kluft C. Evidence for the occurrence of a fast-acting inhibitor for tissue-type plasminogen activator in human plasma. Thromb Haemost 1984; 51: 392–5.
30. Chmielewska JN, Wiman B. Determination of tissue plasminogen activator and its 'fast' inhibitor in plasma. Clin Chem 1986; 32: 482–5.
31. Jespersen J. How to detect defects of tissue plasminogen activator in thrombosis-prone patients. An introduction to discussion. Fibrinolysis 1988; 2/Suppl 2: 104–11.
32. Nguyen G, Horellou MH, Kruithof EKO, Conard J, Samama MM. Residual plasminogen activator inhibitor activity after venous stasis as a criterion for hypofibrinolysis: a study in 83 patients with confirmed deep vein thrombosis. Blood 1988; 72: 601–5.
33. Jennings I, Luddington RJ, Harper PL. Changes in endothelial-related coagulation proteins in response to venous occlusion. Thromb Haemost 1991; 65: 374–6.
34. Keber D. Mechanism of tissue plasminogen activator release during venous occlusion. Fibrinolysis 1988; 2/Suppl 2: 96–103.
35. Petäjä J. Fibrinolytic response to venous occlusion for 10 and 20 minutes in healthy subjects and in patients with deep vein thrombosis. Thromb Res 1989; 56: 251–63.
36. Jespersen J. Gaps between the present assay practice in haemostasis and clinical chemistry laboratories. Fibrinolysis 1990; 4/Suppl 2: 118–20.
37. Nicoloso G, Hauert J, Kruithof EKO, Van Melle G, Bachmann F. Fibrinolysis in normal subjects – comparison between plasminogen activator inhibitor and other components of the fibrinolytic system. Thromb Haemost 1988; 59: 299–303.
38. Sultan Y, Harris A, Strauch G, Venot A, De Lauture D. A dynamic test to investigate potential tissue plasminogen activator activity. Comparison of deamino-8-D-argininevasopressin with venous occlusion in normal subjects and patients. J Lab Clin Med 1988; 111: 645–53.

27
List of manufacturers

Materials and reagents for assays below correspond with the content of the assay chapters and are followed by a list of addresses.

Blood collection and preparation

Diatube 'H' Anticoagulant	Diagnostica Stago
Trombotect anticoagulant (part no. 7203-01)	Abbott Laboratories
Vacutainer tubes (plain, citrate, EDTA, CTAD)	Becton Dickinson
Venoject tubes	Terumo

Antithrombin III activity

Berichrom AT-III	Behringwerke AG
Coatest Antithrombin	KabiVitrum Diagnostica
Stachrom AT-III	Diagnostica Stago
Standard	NIBSC

Antithrombin III antigen

AT III antiserum	Behringwerke AG
Standard	Behringwerke AG
	NIBSC

α_2-Antiplasmin

Control plasma	Behringwerke AG
	Diagnostica Stago
	KabiVitrum Diagnostica
	Organon Teknika
Plasmin	KabiVitrum Diagnostica
Standard (CTS-standard plasma)	Behringwerke AG
Substrate (S-2251)	KabiVitrum Diagnostica

Activated partial thromboplastin time (APTT)
Manchester APTT

UK Reference Laboratory
for Anticoagulant
Reagents and Quality
Control

Bβ 15–42 peptide
Bβ 15–42 peptide (RIA Reagents)

Imco

β-Thromboglobulin
Asserachrom β-TG (ELISA) (cat. no.
DS 0419)
β-Thromboglobulin (RIA) (cat. no. IM-88)
Standard

Diagnostica Stago
Amersham International
NIBSC

Degradation products
D-DIMER

American Diagnostica Inc.
Boehringer Mannheim
GmbH
Diagnostica Stago
MabCo.

Fibrin Degradation Products (FbDP)
Fibrinogen Degradation Products (FgDP)
Total Degradation Products (TDP)

Organon Teknika
Organon Teknika
Organon Teknika

Euglobulin clot lysis time (ECLT)
Bovine Thrombin 5,000 U/vial
(prod. no. NDC 0053-7102-01)
$CaCl_2$ (1 M) analar (prod. no. 19046)
Glacial acetic acid (prod. no. 2789)
TRIS (prod. no. T-3253)

Tween 80 (prod. no. P-1754)

Armour Pharmaceuticals
BDH Chemicals Ltd.
BDH Chemicals Ltd.
Sigma Chemical
Company Ltd.
Sigma Chemical
Company Ltd.

Factor VII clotting activity
Factor VII-deficient plasma

UK Reference Laboratory
for Anticoagulant
Reagents and Quality
Control

Thromborel S (Human Thromboplastin)

Behringwerke AG

Factor VIII clotting activity

Baxter Healthcare
Corporation Dade
Division
Diagnostica Stago
KabiVitrum Diagnostica
Organon Teknika

218

Standard

Ortho Diagnostic Systems
NIBSC

Fibrinogen clotting activity
Reagent

Baxter Dade AG
Behringwerke AG
BioMérieux
Diagnostica Stago

Standard — NIBSC

Fibrinopeptide A (FPA)
Asserachrom FPA — Diagnostica Stago
Imco FPA (RIA) — Imco
RIA-mat FPA — Altana Inc.
Byk-Sangtec Diagnostica

Histidine-rich glycoprotein (HRG)
Agarose Litex HSA — FMC Bioproducts
Barbituric Acid — Merck
Heparin (Porcine mucosa) — Leo Pharmaceuticals
HRG antiserum — Behringwerke AG
Sodium Barbiturate — Merck
Tris — Sigma Chemical Company Ltd.

Platelet factor 4 (PF4)
Asserachrom PF4 (ELISA) (cat. no. DS 0414) — Diagnostica Stago
PF4 Enzygnost (ELISA) — Behringwerke AG
PF4-RIA (part. no. 7856-24) — Abbott Laboratories
Standard — NIBSC

Plasmin–α_2-antiplasmin complexes (PAP-complexes)
PAP-kits (ELISA) — Technoclone Inc.
Teijin Ltd.

Plasminogen activity
Plasminogen standard (glu-plasminogen) — NIBSC
Streptase — Behringwerke AG
Streptokinase — KabiVitrum Diagnostica
Substrate Chromozym PL — Boehringer Mannheim
Substrate S-2251 — KabiVitrum Diagnostica

Plasminogen activator inhibitor activity
Kits and reagents

American Diagnostics
Behringwerke AG
Biopool AB
Diagnostica Stago
KabiVitrum Diagnostica

Plasminogen activator inhibitor antigen
Imulyse PAI-1 (ELISA) — Biopool AB
TintElize PAI-1 (ELISA) — Biopool AB
PAI:Ag (ELISA) — American Diagnostics
Monozyme
Technoclone Inc.

Protein C activity
Coa-set Protein C — KabiVitrum Diagnostica

Protein C antigen
ELISA — Diagnostica Stago
Organon Teknika
Laurell (plates) — American Diagnostics
Diagnostica Stago

Laurell (reagents)
Agarose IndubioseA-37 — Pharma-Industrie IBF
Agarose T — Behringwerke AG
Barbital — Merck
EDTA — Boehringer Mannheim GmbH

Gelbond film — FMC Bioproducts
Seakem LE Agarose — FMC Bioproducts
Sodium Barbital — Merck
Tris — Sigma Chemical Company Ltd.

Protein S antigen
Asserachrom Protein S (ELISA) — Diagnostica Stago
Laurell — American Diagnostics
Diagnostica Stago

Prothrombin time test (PT)
Manchester Reagent thromboplastin — UK Reference Laboratory for Anticoagulant Reagents and Quality Control

Tissue-type plasminogen activator activity
Kits and reagents — American Diagnostics
Biopool AB
Boehringer Mannheim GmbH
Diagnostica Stago
KabiVitrum Diagnostica
Organon Teknika
Standard — NIBSC

Tissue-type plasminogen activator antigen

Asserachrom t-PA (ELISA)	Diagnostica Stago
Coaliza t-PA (ELISA)	KabiVitrum Diagnostica
Imulyse t-PA (ELISA)	Biopool AB
Innotest t-PA (ELISA)	Innogenetics NV
Standard	NIBSC
TintElize t-PA (ELISA)	Biopool AB
t-PA assay kit (ELISA)	Cabru
	Imco
	Monozyme

Thrombin–antithrombin III complexes (TAT-complexes)

Enzygnost TAT (ELISA)	Behringwerke AG

von Willebrand factor

Asserachrom vWF (ELISA)	Diagnostica Stago
VonWF:Ag (ELISA)	American Diagnostics
Standard	NIBSC

ADDRESSES

Abbott Laboratories
Diagnostic Division
Abbott House, Moorbridge Road
Maidenhead, Berks. SL6 8XN
United Kingdom
Tel: +44 628 78 40 41
Fax: +44 628 34 866

Altana Inc.
60 Baylis Road
Melville, NY 11747
USA
Tel: +1 516 454 76 77

American Diagnostics
222 Railroad Avenue
P.O. Box 1165
Greenwich CT 06836-1165
USA
Tel: +1 203 661 0000
Fax: +1 203 661 77 84

Amersham International plc
Lincoln Place, Green End
Aylesbury, Bucks. HP 20 2TP
United Kingdom
Tel: +44 296 39 522
Fax: +44 296 85 910

Armour Pharmaceuticals
Saint Leonard's House
Saint Leonard's Road
Eastbourne
East Sussex
United Kingdom
Tel: +44 323 41 02 00
Fax: +44 323 41 03 06

Bayer AG
D-5090 Leverkussen
Bagerwerk
Germany
Tel: +49 214 301
Fax: +49 214 3066 411

Baxter Dade AG
Bonnstrasse 9
CH-3186 Düdingen
Switzerland
Tel: +41 37 43 81 11
Fax: +41 37 43 89 60

Baxter Healthcare Corporation
Brand Facility
550 North Brand Boulevard
Glendale CA 91203
USA
Tel: +1 818 956 32 00
Fax: +1 818 507 55 96

BDH Chemicals Limited
Fourways
Carylon Industrial Estate
Atherstone
Warwickshire
CV9 1GJ
United Kingdom
Tel: +44 827 71 77 66
Fax: +44 827 71 88 44

Becton Dickinson
Immunocytometry Systems
2350 Qume Drive, San José
CA 95131-1807
USA
Tel: +1 800 223 82 26
Fax: +1 408 954 20 09

Behringwerke AG
P.O. Box 1140
D-3550 Marburg 1
Germany
Tel: +49 642 13 94 494
Fax: +49 642 13 13 88

BioMérieux
Marcy – l'Etoile
69260 Charbonnières-les-Bains
France
Tel: +33 16 (7) 887 8110
Fax: +33 337 88 720 90

Biopool AB
Box 1454
S-901 24 Umeå
Sweden
Tel: +46 90 19 00 00
Fax: +46 90 19 45 00

Boehringer Mannheim GmbH
Biochemica
Sandhofer Strasse 116
Postfach 31 0120
D-6800 Mannheim 31
Germany
Tel: +49 621 75 91
Fax: +49 621 75 98 509

Byk-Sangtec Diagnostica
von Hevesy-Strasse
D-6057 Dietzenbach 2
Germany
Tel: +49 60 74 401 0
Fax: +49 60 74 401 209

Cabru
Via Caduti per la Patria, 47
20050 Peregallo di Lesmo
Italy
Tel: +39 698 15 89
Fax: +39 606 51 74

Diagnostica Stago
6ter Rue Denis Papin
F-92600 Asnières sur Seine
France
Tel: +33 1 47 33 40 60
Fax: +33 1 34 15 47 79

FMC Corporation Bioproducts
5 Maple Street
Rockland ME 04841-2994
USA
Tel: +1 207 594 3200

Imco
Hudiksvallsgatan 4B
S-113 30 Stockholm
Sweden
Tel: +46 8 33 53 09
Fax: +46 8 728 47 76

Innogenetics NV
Kronenbrugstraat 45
2000 Antwerpen
Belgium
Tel: +32 3 216 4820
Fax: +32 323 216 44 97

KabiVitrum Diagnostica
Taljegardsgatan 3
S-43 153 Mölndal
Sweden
Tel: +46 31 27 52 40
Fax: +46 31 86 46 26

MabCo
P.O. Box 475
Springwood Old 4127
Australia

Leo Pharmaceuticals
Industrivej 55
DK-2750 Ballerup
Denmark
Tel: +45 44 94 58 88
Fax: +45 44 94 30 40

E. Merck Darmstadt
Postfach 4119
D-6100 Damstadt
Frankfurter Strasse 250
Germany
Tel: +49 06151 720
Fax: +49 06151 72 33 68

Monozyme
Søbakken 15
DK-2920 Charlottenlund
Denmark
Tel: +45 31 64 13 38
Fax: +45 31 64 14 89

National Institute for
Biological Standards and Control
Blanche Lane
South Mimms
Potters Bar
Hertfordshire EN6 3QG
United Kingdom
Tel: +44 707 54 753
Fax: +44 707 46 730

Organon Teknika
Veedijk 58
2300 Turnhout
Belgium
Tel: +32 14 40 40 40
Fax: +32 14 42 16 00

Ortho Diagnostic Systems Inc.
US Route 202
Ratitan 08869 N.J.
USA
Tel: +1 201 524 23 74

Pharma-Industrie IBF
35 Avenue Jean Jaurès
92390 Villeneuve – La Garennes
France
Tel: +33 1 46 85 92 00
Fax: +33 1 47 92 26 55

Sigma Chemical Company Ltd.
Fancy Road
Poole
Dorset
BH17 7NH
United Kingdom
Tel: +44 202 73 31 14
Fax: +44 202 71 54

Technoclone Inc.
Müllnergasse 23
A-1090 Vienna
Austria
Tel: +43 1 34 22 80 or +43 1 34 23 22
Fax: +43 1 31 52 78

Teijin Ltd.
Uchisaiwai-cho 2-1-1
Chiyoda-ku
Tokyo 100
Japan
Tel: +81 3 35 06 48 92
Fax: +81 3 35 08 27 67

Terumo Corporation
Interleuvenlaan 40
3001 Leuven
Belgium
Tel: +32 16 38 12 11
Fax: +32 16 22 91 04

The Immunoassay Kit Directory

Editor:

John Seth, *University of Edinburgh, UK*

The Immunoassay Kit Directory is a comprehensive, independent and up-to-date reference source of the many commercially available immunoassay kits in use by clinical chemists, biochemists, and endocrinologists.

Each kit is described in detail, over 20 different major parameters being listed in a consistent manner to allow for easy comparison.

Key facts are provided, including: Assay type, sample type and number of tests; Antibodies and antigens used; Detection system; No of stage and time taken; Special equipment and reagents needed; Standards used; Sensitivity, specificity and precision; Limitations and expected values;

New for 1992

KLUWER ACADEMIC PUBLISHERS

Subscription Information ISSN 0926-2067
1991/92, Volume 1 (4 issues)
Subscription rate Dfl. 650.00/US$395.00
incl. postage/handling

P.O. Box 322, 3300 AH Dordrecht, The Netherlands
P.O. Box 358, Accord Station, Hingham, MA 02018-0358, U.S.A.

Index

225